Praise for *Prevent a Second Heart Attack*

"Dr. Brill provides an engaging and informative book for patients and providers alike. This exceptional book provides easy-to-read information on nutrition and heart disease, practical approaches to heart healthy living, and tools to help patients successfully reduce heart-disease risk. I will recommend this book most highly to all my patients."

—JoAnne M. Foody, M.D., FACC, FAHA, medical director
of Cardiovascular Wellness at Brigham and Women's Hospital

"For the thirteen million Americans who have survived a heart attack or are diagnosed with heart disease, this book is a MUST read! In [a] thorough, thoughtful, evidence-based, user-friendly approach, Dr. Brill presents the eight key foods and lifestyle changes needed to CONQUER heart disease. This book provides the roadmap to successfully navigating the way to a long healthy life after a heart attack."

—Jennifer H. Mieres, M.D., FACC, FAHA, cardiologist,
coauthor of *Heart Smart for Black Women and Latinas*

"A superb resource for health professionals and consumers! Dr. Brill covers it all! I will recommend her book wholeheartedly to my patients who want science-based guidelines to keep their hearts healthy naturally with nutritious foods and exercise."

—Georgia Kostas, MPH, RD, LD, author of
The Cooper Clinic Solution to the Diet Revolution

Also by Janet Brill

Cholesterol Down

PREVENT A SECOND HEART ATTACK

8 Foods, 8 Weeks
to Reverse Heart Disease

Janet Bond Brill, Ph.D., R.D., LDN

Foreword by **Annabelle S. Volgman,** M.D., F.A.C.C.

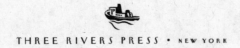

THREE RIVERS PRESS • NEW YORK

This book is not intended as a replacement for qualified and professional medical care. Individuals with diagnosed cardiovascular disease and/or those at risk for cardiovascular disease should first consult with their personal physician for medical clearance before making any of the dietary and lifestyle changes recommended in *Prevent a Second Heart Attack*. The Prevent a Second Heart Attack plan should not be followed without the express permission of your personal physician. Although several versions of the Mediterranean diet have been scientifically proven to lower the risk of death from a recurrent cardiovascular event, the Prevent a Second Heart Attack plan, outlined in this book, has not yet been scientifically shown to do so. Although every effort has been made to provide accurate and up-to-date information, this document cannot be guaranteed to be free of factual error. All of the recommendations set forth in these pages are supported by research; however, many are based on observational studies. Observational studies are not the gold standard of research known as randomized clinical trials, so although the cause and effect cannot be definitively established, in many instances the association and potential health benefits can be. Consult your physician regarding applicability of any information provided in this book for your medical condition. Furthermore, both the author and the publisher take no responsibility for any consequences that may arise from following the advice set forth within these pages.

Copyright © 2011 by Janet Brill, Ph.D.

All rights reserved.

Published in the United States by Three Rivers Press, an imprint of the Crown Publishing Group, a division of Random House, Inc., New York.

www.crownpublishing.com

Three Rivers Press and the Tugboat design are registered trademarks of Random House, Inc.

Library of Congress Cataloging-in-Publication

Brill, Janet Bond.
    Prevent a second heart attack : 8 foods, 8 weeks to reverse heart disease / Janet Bond Brill.—1st ed.
        p.   cm.
    Includes bibliographical references and index.
    ISBN 978-0-307-46525-2
    1. Heart—Diseases—Prevention—Popular works.   2. Heart—Diseases—Diet therapy—Recipes.   I. Title.
    RC672.B683 2011
    616.1'2—dc 22   2010038490

Printed in the United States of America

Illustrations on pages 30, 31, 36, 40, 42, 45, and 48 by Mia Alexandra Brill

10 9 8 7 6 5 4 3 2 1

First Edition

To my husband, Sam, whom I adore . . . may you outlive me.

To my father, Rudy Bond, I miss you, Daddy.

To my brother, Zane Philip Bond, I miss you too, Zippy.

To my beautiful children, Rachel, Mia, and Jason:
I am a writer, I am a nutritionist, I am a friend,
I am a daughter, and I am a wife, but first and foremost,
I am your mother—and nothing at all would be
worth anything to me without all of you.

Contents

Section 3: Stay Active: Movement = Heart Health

Part III: THE PREVENT A SECOND HEART ATTACK PLAN IN ACTION

Section 1: 14-Day Meal Plan

Section 2: Recipes

Foreword

Many women come up to me after hearing one of my lectures and tell me they want to be my patient after their first heart attack. I warn them in the gentlest way possible that they may not survive their first heart attack. Thirty percent of first heart attacks result in sudden cardiac death. These people never even make it to the hospital. A recent famous example is Tim Russert, the beloved *Meet the Press* anchorman.

To prevent a heart attack, it's not enough to take medications. A whole package of lifestyle changes is needed, including the foods you eat and the physical activities you pursue.

Dr. Janet Bond Brill's new book, *Prevent a Second Heart Attack*, can help prevent a second heart attack and prevent a first one from happening.

This is the take-home book for heart attack survivors.

After a heart attack, most patients receive a visit from a dietitian who provides a list of foods to embrace and foods to avoid. A heart attack is a wake-up call. It's a good time to learn about changing diet and lifestyle. But back home, it is easy to slip back into bad habits. This book is something patients can read to understand why they need to change their diet.

Indeed, this book is an excellent source of information for any heart disease patient, not just people who have had a heart attack. Dr. Brill teaches us what a heart-healthy diet is and why foods such as fish, olive oil, fruits and vegetables—even chocolate—can reverse heart disease.

As a cardiologist I see patients every day who need to be educated about lifestyle changes. The way they've been living has made them ill or unhealthy with obesity, high blood pressure, high cholesterol, or diabetes. When I opened the Rush Heart Center for Women in 2003, the first of its kind in Chicago, I made sure we had nutritionists available to all our patients, free of charge, because most of our patients needed advice about the foods they eat and the exercise they undertake.

For most patients, it seems hard to believe that their doctors aren't experts in nutrition. Wouldn't they know what kinds of foods heart disease patients should or shouldn't be eating? Doctors tell patients to eat a heart-healthy diet and assume that patients know what that is. Many cardiologists still recommend a bland low-fat diet. Most patients don't realize that doctors are not educated in any significant way about nutrition. Medical schools cover basic physiology, anatomy, pharmacology, and diseases. Until I started the Rush Heart Center for Women, I, too, had very little knowledge of heart-healthy nutrition. I turned to my colleagues in the nutrition department, who taught me well and continue to share new findings with me.

I was so certain that lifestyle was the key to heart health, I considered going back to school to get a degree in nutrition!

Reading Dr. Brill's writings has become part of my ongoing education.

What I love about this new book is that it says yes to the pleasure of food, unlike the Ornish and Pritikin diets. Dr. Brill makes a heart-healthy diet a feast for the eyes, nose, and palate. She recommends the most colorful, beautiful, and delicious foods the earth has to offer, which nourish our bodies. The recipes in the back are a great way of incorporating all the foods mentioned in the book.

Why food? Why not supplements? Study after study has shown that antioxidant vitamins such as A, B, C, and E help prevent "bad" cholesterol from becoming toxic to the arteries. At the same time, these vitamins, when taken as supplements, slightly increase major cardiovascular events or cancers. What are we to believe? Should doctors tell their patients to stop taking vitamins?

This is what we've learned: Vitamins that are essential to life (after all, vitamins are *vital amines*) have to come from whole foods. Not from a tablet. Vitamins are indeed essential for life, but they have to be bought in the produce section of the store, not in the bottled vitamin section.

From Dr. Brill, I've learned that a daily dose of leafy green vegetables can markedly decrease one's risk of developing diabetes. She also showed me the scientific evidence that eating three or more servings of fruit daily significantly decreases the risk of a heart attack.

I read Dr. Brill's brilliant first book, *Cholesterol Down*, out loud, word for word, to my husband, who had just been diagnosed with high cholesterol. We both learned that taking statins isn't enough to prevent a first heart attack or stroke. We had to make the switch to a heart-healthy lifestyle. I only wish Tim Russert had known that, too.

The message in this book is clear: Eating heart-healthy foods and being physically active is your body's best medicine. Read this to prevent your second heart attack or stroke. Pass it on to someone you care about to prevent his or her first.

I truly believe that the *Brill* in Dr. Brill's name is short for *Brilliant!* Bravo, Janet, on another masterpiece. Thank you from the bottom of my heart—the endothelial layer of our arteries.

—ANNABELLE S. VOLGMAN, M.D., FACC
Medical Director, Rush Heart Center for Women
Associate Professor
Rush University Medical Center
Chicago, Illinois

Acknowledgments

I could not have written this book without the help of so many of my professional colleagues, friends, and family. Thank you all for your support and for helping me to scale a great mountain that for me was truly one of the greatest accomplishments of my life.

To my mother, Dr. Alma Bond, thanks for all of your support and for showing me that women can do it all . . . write books, teach, work, be a good wife and a great mom. And to my "other" parents, Harry and Edna Brill, you are kindhearted, good, generous people. I am so fortunate to have you as my "other" parents. I love you very much and, by the way, thank you for your son!

This manuscript could not have been compiled without the help of my longtime editor extraordinaire, Jody Berman. Thank you, Jody, for polishing up my diamond in the rough and also for your superb attention to detail and incredible speed, which once again allowed me to make that looming deadline. Heartfelt thanks to my lovely new editor at Three Rivers Press, Anna Thompson. Anna, you are truly a joy to work with and your editing skills are the best in the business. My gratitude is also extended to my other two editors at Random House, Emily Timberlake and Lindsay Orman, both of whom sadly moved on during my initial book-writing process. I would especially like to acknowledge my agent, Faith Hamlin. Once again, thank you, Faith, for having the confidence in me to write a second book. I appreciate your relentless support and guidance.

To Maggie Green, a phenomenal chef and a registered dietitian all-in-one. Thank you, thank you, thank you for all your help with testing most and developing many of the recipes—you are as good as it gets for a top-notch professional. Much gratitude to all the chefs who were so kind to share with me and the world your mouth-watering and superbly heart-healthy creations.

To my highly esteemed colleague Annabelle Volgman, M.D., thank you for writing the wonderfully informative forward to this book. I greatly appreciate your valuable contribution to this project and as always I look forward to having the opportunity to share the speaking stage with such a lovely person and a true pioneer in the field of women's heart health.

I would like to extend my heartfelt thanks to all my friends who were there for me during this long process of writing. To our spectacular personal trainer, Vladimir Magloire, thank you for everything and especially thank you for your wonderful friendship. For all of our dear friends who supported me during my husband's nightmarish heart attack scenario—I don't know what I would have done without you (this means *you,* Brian and Lynn Berkowitz). Oh, and Dr. Simkins, thanks for saving my husband's life!

PREVENT A SECOND HEART ATTACK

Introduction

My father had a heart attack when he was forty-five. Twenty years later he had a second heart attack—the one that killed him. Sadly, he was given no lifestyle advice that could have prevented that second and fatal event. My own husband, Sam, had a heart attack—his first—on July 31, 2009, and thankfully he survived with minimal damage to his heart muscle. Fearful that he would suffer my father's fate, I chose to write this book for him, to help him live a long, healthy and happy life, despite his heart disease diagnosis—to teach him and other heart patients how to prevent that second, lethal attack and even reverse the actual disease process. But perhaps more important, I wanted to give hope to all of those who have suffered through the trauma of a heart attack: to tell them that the ideal heart-healthy diet is *not* one of deprivation, but rather a deliciously palatable Mediterranean style of living that will enable them to enjoy eating—one of life's greatest pleasures. *Prevent a Second Heart Attack* does just that.

If you are reading this book, chances are that you or a loved one has had a heart attack. Having a heart attack used to be a death sentence. Today that is no longer the case. But this book is not just about helping you prevent a repeat attack; it is also about how to live *well* with heart disease. A heart disease diagnosis doesn't mean that you have to give up all that you enjoy in life. Most heart

---

A NATION OF HEART-DISEASE-PRONE BABY BOOMERS

Currently some 26.6 million Americans have survived a heart attack or have been diagnosed with heart disease. "Heart disease deaths are projected to increase sharply between 2010 and 2030, and the population of heart disease survivors is expected to grow at a much faster rate than the U.S. population as a whole." We are a population of aging, heart-disease-prone baby boomers. In fact, "people 75 and older are the fastest-growing segment of the population, and 40 percent of them have heart disease."

Sources: Centers for Disease Control and Prevention, Division for Heart Disease and Stroke Prevention, "A public health action plan to prevent heart disease and stroke," http://www .cdc.gov/dhdsp/library/action_plan/full_sec1_scope_burden.htm; Centers for Disease Control and Prevention, "FastStats," http://www.cdc.gov/nchs/fastats/heart.htm; and "Good survival rates found in heart surgery for aged," *New York Times,* November 11, 2008.

---

patients can lead happy, healthy lives—without the hardship of following a tasteless, low-fat, or highly restrictive diet. Advances in medical research and technology have proven that there is a much better way for heart attack survivors to prevent new plaque buildup and stabilize and even reverse dangerous, vulnerable plaque in their coronary arteries and the new way is a delightful, appetizing diet and lifestyle plan. The Prevent a Second Heart Attack plan is *not* a bland, low-fat diet, but rather a simple and delicious Mediterranean-style eating strategy based on clinically tested research that proves that this method can cut the risk of a second heart attack by up to 70 percent!

WHY FOCUS ON A SECOND HEART ATTACK?

As a registered dietitian specializing in cardiovascular disease prevention, I have found a great need among heart attack survivors that is not being met. These are the people who are the most receptive to making lifestyle changes to reduce the risk of a second heart attack. Having a brush with death bestows powerful motivation to do what it takes to live—and hopefully to prevent that second and potentially fatal cardiac event. Yet the lifestyle message is not getting through to some of these individuals.

Unfortunately, many heart attack survivors are not receiving preventive lifestyle advice from their cardiologists. After enduring severe physical, psychological, and emotional duress, some patients are handed difficult and perplexing dietary guidelines for heart-healthy eating. Others are given no lifestyle advice at all. Cardiologists often do not have the time to advise their patients, and patients may not want to pay the additional cost for counseling from registered dietitians, which often is not covered by their insurance.

Despite being highly motivated to change their lifestyle, the *large majority* (some 80 percent) of patients with heart disease fail to adhere to dietary advice one year after their diagnosis.[1] Why? When asked, patients cite *confusion* as the main reason for their lack of compliance. Furthermore, these same researchers have shown that "keeping the message simple is the key to improving dietary advice to patients." This valuable research pinpoints where most post–heart attack patients go wrong in their eating regimen: Many avoid carbs and thus get little heart-healthy fiber; most consume excessive amounts of harmful sodium and trans fats; and few get in the disease-reversing, phytonutrient-rich vegetables and fruits that are key to preventing a second heart attack. Patients want to comply, but they need clear, doable options if they are to change their diet and prevent their disease from progressing. *Prevent a Second Heart Attack* does just that—and goes a step further, offering straightforward lifestyle advice that is scientifically proven to prevent a second heart attack *and* reverse the disease process.

THE PROOF IS IN THE SCIENTIFIC PUDDING

As many as half a million Americans will die of heart disease this year, making coronary heart disease the single largest killer of men

> ## SOBERING STATISTICS
>
> According to the American Heart Association, each year approximately
>
> - 785,000 Americans will have a new heart attack
> - 470,000 will have a recurrent attack
> - 195,000 individuals will experience an additional silent heart attack
>
> In other words, roughly 1.5 million people will have a heart attack this year (that's the size of the entire population of the state of Rhode Island). Thirty-eight percent of them (more than half a million Americans) will die from it. That means 62 percent will survive and must learn to live with the diagnosis of heart disease and the perpetual anxiety of possibly having another attack.
>
> Source: American Heart Association, *Heart Disease and Stroke Statistics—2010 Update* (Dallas, TX: American Heart Association, 2010).

and women in the United States.[2] What has the scientific community provided us in terms of proven steps to help reverse this situation?

Overwhelming scientific evidence shows that more that 80 percent of heart attacks can be prevented in both women and men through lifestyle factors. This is as true for individuals who have never had a diagnosis of heart disease as for those who have already had a heart attack. The latest research shows that post–heart attack patients should follow this general lifestyle advice:

1. Eat a heart-healthy diet.

2. Practice healthful stress management.

3. Be physically active.

4. Don't smoke.

5. Achieve a healthy weight.

6. Take medications.[3]

What, then, are the *best* diet and exercise changes—when partnered with doctor-prescribed drugs—that this population should make to prevent repeat attacks? This is the very question that this book will answer. There is a tremendous amount of scientific research to draw from, and the research shows that my simplified Mediterranean lifestyle (diet, exercise, and stress management) is the optimal lifestyle plan for preventing a second heart attack, halting heart disease, and even promoting regression. In fact, the famed Lyon Heart Study tested a Cretan Mediterranean diet in cardiac patients and proved in its clinical research that this lifestyle cuts the risk of a second attack by a phenomenal 50 to 70 percent when compared to heart patients following a typical low-fat American Heart Association–style diet.[4] The scientific evidence is crystal clear: This lifestyle prescription is far superior to the low-fat regimens typically prescribed to heart patients in the fat-phobic 1990s (regimens that continue to fill the heart disease section of bookstore shelves).

BREAKTHROUGH THERAPEUTIC LIFESTYLE APPROACH

Prevent a Second Heart Attack crystallizes what researchers have termed the gold standard for cardiovascular disease prevention—the Mediterranean diet—into a simple, accessible nutrition plan for heart disease reversal. It explains how eight specific foods (including olive oil and omega-3-rich fish such as salmon), when eaten in combination, have spectacular heart benefits—such as preventing plaque buildup and even stabilizing or reversing plaque in the coronary arteries—with scientific support explaining why.

Several heart disease reversal books currently available in bookstores advocate spartan, vegan-style plans that are either too difficult to follow or just not livable. (One recommends twenty different supplements in addition to diet, several of which have been proven ineffective in preventing cardiovascular disease!)

General heart disease prevention books offer volumes of information about the primary prevention of heart disease, and some offer general concepts for reversing heart disease, but none specifically targets *the second heart attack,* until now.

HOW TO USE THIS BOOK

Within these pages, you will find a *simple,* easy-to-follow lifestyle (diet and exercise) plan designed to help heart attack survivors achieve longer and fuller lives. There are three main parts to this book:

• Part I (Chapters 1–3) provides an in-depth scientific background and is useful for those individuals seeking to understand the nuts and bolts of their disease and the logic behind the preventive steps in *Prevent a Second Heart Attack.* For example, Chapter 2 addresses the science of atherosclerosis—the underlying cause of heart attacks—and translates the often confusing science into clear and understandable language. However, if this section is too scientific for your taste, feel free to skip ahead to the diet section and start today to protect yourself against a second heart attack.

• Part II (Chapters 4–14) is the diet and exercise lifestyle section. This part of the book includes step-by-step guidelines for eating the highly palatable Mediterranean way, including food prescriptions (eight daily and weekly food groups) and an exercise plan, as well as the most recent scientific rationale supporting the recommendations.

• Part III includes fourteen days of meal plans accompanied by more than fifty Mediterranean-inspired recipes, many contributed by top chefs. These recipes are easy to cook, delicious, and healthy, and include nutritional analyses. In addition, the Appendix contains a helpful lifestyle prescription daily checklist, which is an extremely valuable tool that will help you stick to the plan.

GETTING MAXIMUM CARDIO PROTECTION

For anyone, with or without diagnosed heart disease, interested in the ideal comprehensive heart disease prevention or reversal plan, I suggest using this book in combination with my previous book, *Cholesterol Down* (Crown/Three Rivers Press). This will enable you to get your "bad" LDL cholesterol under control using several foods specified in *Cholesterol Down,* as well as provide you with the full background diet and lifestyle plan outlined in this book to ameliorate other heart disease risk factors. Although the ten steps in *Cholesterol Down* would certainly benefit all individuals as a first step in preventing heart disease, for those with heart disease—who *must* keep their LDL, or "bad" cholesterol, under control—focusing on just LDL cholesterol is not enough. Heart disease survivors with LDL cholesterol controlled by medication (and I would hope diet) need to follow a much more complete lifestyle plan—in conjunction with medications—to up the odds of warding off a second heart attack.

For the millions of Americans living with heart disease, *Prevent a Second Heart Attack* presents a tasty, easy-to-follow set of lifestyle guidelines based on the phenomenally heart-healthy and delicious Mediterranean style of eating. Holding this book in your hands, mind, and heart not only leads to huge health gains; it could potentially save your life. Read on, and start today maximizing your defenses against that second heart attack—while learning to slow down, enjoy food, and live a longer, healthier life. À votre santé!

Part I

How You Got Heart Disease in the First Place

1

Making the Transition from Sickness to Health

The gods are just, and of our pleasant vices

Make instruments to plague us.

—*King Lear,* William Shakespeare (1564–1616)

Why are so many people having heart attacks in the United States? What triggers the formation of that first "fatty streak"—the earliest visible hint that something is awry in the arteries—and the eventual onset of advanced heart disease (a.k.a. atherosclerotic cardiovascular disease), our nation's leading killer?

We used to think that heart attacks were an inevitable consequence of aging. But in the last decades, research has revealed a surprising truth: Heart disease is a lifestyle-borne illness, and atherosclerosis (the leading cause of heart attacks and stroke, and the defining term for when fatty deposits build up inside the arterial walls) begins in childhood. A toxic mix of calorie overload, especially of processed foods high in damaging fats, sugars, and salt, coupled with inactivity instigates the long, slow process of arterial damage that results in a heart attack.

In this chapter, you will discover how, when, and why your own coronary arteries began to clog up, thereby setting the stage for atherosclerotic cardiovascular disease. You will learn about how you can take control of your heart health the Prevent a Second Heart Attack way—a doable strategy allowing you to take action to switch your disease course and ultimately remain a "survivor" for many decades to come.

BASIC HEART ATTACK FACTS

• A heart attack is also known as a "myocardial infarction."

• A heart attack occurs when the blood supply flowing through the arteries that feed the heart (a.k.a. the coronary arteries) is cut off, resulting in damage or death in part of the heart muscle.

• Blockage in the coronary artery is generally caused by severe arterial damage, the result of years of plaque buildup in the artery walls, a progressive disease process called *atherosclerosis.*

• Atherosclerosis occurs when plaque builds up in the coronary arteries, the pipes that feed the heart muscle, which is why you will hear doctors refer to the disease as *coronary artery disease* (CAD).

• Heart attacks are the primary cause of death of American men and women; every twenty-five seconds, an American will suffer a heart attack, and once a minute someone will die from one.

• About one sixth of all heart attacks are "silent," meaning the person who has one is unaware it takes place; silent heart attacks can damage the heart muscle.

• Occasionally, a blockage in a coronary artery causes a disturbance in the electrical rhythm of the heart; this is called an *arrhythmia* and can cause sudden death.

• A healthy lifestyle can reduce the risk of a heart attack by as much as 92 percent.

Sources: American Heart Association, *Heart Disease and Stroke Statistics—2010 Update* (Dallas, TX: American Heart Association, 2010); and Agneta Akesson et al., "Combined effect of low-risk dietary and lifestyle behaviors in primary prevention of myocardial infarction in women," *Archives of Internal Medicine* 167, no. 19 (2007): 2122–2127.

YOU ARE WHAT YOU EAT

It is well known that what you eat and your level of physical activity have a major impact on your health. A poor diet greatly increases your risk of developing any number of chronic health conditions and diseases, including high blood pressure, obesity, diabetes, osteoporosis, several types of cancer, and heart disease.

Researchers at the University of North Carolina School of Medicine conducted a survey study examining the nutritional habits and chronic indicators of disease in 1,788 men and women whose average age was forty-eight.[1] They found that people who ate a poor diet had significantly higher rates of disease (such as those with diagnosed high blood pressure and/or heart disease). A poor diet was also strongly associated with individuals at high risk of contracting a chronic disease precursor such as prediabetes. What type of diet did the high-risk people eat? One that was loaded with fast-food meals, sugary drinks, high-fat snacks, and lots of desserts/sweets; low in fruits and vegetables; and coupled with a sedentary lifestyle. The bottom line is, both the type and quantity of food consumed have a profound effect on your risk for heart disease, as diet plays a large role in your resistance or susceptibility to atherosclerosis.[2]

WESTERN DIET PROMOTES HEART ATTACKS

According to a global study of dietary patterns, the best diet for clogging the arteries and promoting heart attacks is the "Western" style of eating. The INTERHEART study looked at 5,761 heart attack cases (taken from subjects in fifty-two countries) and compared the diet of those individuals with the diet of 10,646 people without known heart disease (the control group). The researchers concluded that 30 percent of the risk of heart disease was related to a "poor diet," what they called a Western style of eating, defined as higher intake of fried foods, salty snacks, eggs, and meat. On closer examination of the dietary risk score, a higher score (meaning a poorer diet) was associated with as much as a 92 percent increase in risk of having a heart attack.

Source: Romaina Iqbal et al., "Dietary patterns and the risk of acute myocardial infarction in 52 countries: Results of the INTERHEART Study," *Circulation* 118 (2008): 1929–1937.

What would happen if we took an entire population that for centuries subsisted on a traditional, mostly vegetarian, whole-foods diet and a highly active lifestyle (in which the residents grew their own food) and switched them over to a highly processed, calorie-dense, Western diet and sedentary existence? Researchers in Mexico observed such a phenomenon.[3]

HEART DISEASE RISK FACTORS

The more risk factors you have, and the higher the level of each risk factor, the greater your risk for having both a first heart attack *and a second.* Control of risk factors is crucial for preventing progression of and reversing heart disease. Some risk factors such as age, gender, and family history are *unmodifiable*—in other words, not under your control. Others are considered *modifiable,* and you can take action to change them, a move that will significantly increase your odds for survival.

Major risk factors. Major, established risk factors are those that have a substantial body of scientific evidence showing that they significantly increase risk of heart disease. According to the American Heart Association (AHA), there are six major, treatable risk factors for heart disease:

- High blood cholesterol (especially high levels of low-density lipoprotein cholesterol, or LDL)
- Cigarette smoking
- Diabetes
- High blood pressure
- Overweight/obesity
- Physical inactivity

The World Health Organization (WHO) has added a seventh major risk factor: an unhealthy diet low in fruits and vegetables and high in saturated fat. The WHO also expands and more precisely defines cholesterol. It considers "abnormal blood lipids" (high LDL, low HDL [high-density lipoprotein cholesterol], and a high triglyceride level) a major modifiable risk factor for heart disease.

Contributing, or "other," risk factors. Additional factors have been linked to an increased risk for the development of heart disease, yet their significance does not have enough scientific evidence to classify them as major. According to both the AHA and the WHO, these include the following:

- Chronic and excessive stress
- Heavy alcohol use
- Use of certain medications such as hormone replacement therapy or oral contraceptives
- Mental illness
- Low socioeconomic status
- Lipoprotein (a)—a type of blood fat

Sources: American Heart Association, http://www.americanheart.org/presenter.jhtml?identifier =500, and World Health Organization, http://www.who.int/cardiovascular_diseases/en/cvd _atlas_03_risk_factors.pdf.

The Tepehuanos Indians living in the Sierra Madre Occidental Mountains of northwest Mexico subsisted on a plant-based diet, filled with green vegetables, beans, potatoes, breads, and tortillas made from root vegetables, eating meat and animal products very rarely. In 1995–1996 researchers also found that obesity was rare and diabetes was virtually nonexistent among the Tepehuanos.

In the year 2000, as part of a social assistance program, Western-style foods were made available to the Tepehuanos either for free or at a very low cost. The traditional Tepehuanos diet was thus substantially modified by the introduction of a Western-style diet filled with highly processed salty foods, meat, eggs, sugar, refined flour products, soft drinks, and other types of junk food. The effect of this drastic dietary change was documented at the ten-year follow-up assessment of the study. Total calorie intake rose 42 percent, accompanied by a doubling of protein and artery-clogging saturated fat intake. In addition, there was a notable decline in fiber and carbohydrate intake, as well as a dramatic reduction in the consumption of healthful polyunsaturated fat. The occurrence of heart disease risk factors escalated, mirroring the dietary changes. Obesity, diabetes, high blood pressure, a high blood level of triglycerides, and a low HDL cholesterol value all were now commonplace among the Tepehuanos Indians.

IT ALL BEGINS IN CHILDHOOD

For more than sixty years we have known that atherosclerosis starts in childhood and progresses to cause heart disease in middle age and beyond.[4] Autopsy studies of the hearts of our nation's youth show that atherosclerosis, the underlying cause of CAD, manifests early in life. The 1953 results of an autopsy study of U.S. soldiers (average age twenty-two) killed in the Korean War surprised the nation when it was revealed that 77 percent of the hearts examined showed signs of atherosclerosis.[5] A similar study of U.S. casualties of the Vietnam War showed that 45 percent of the hearts had atherosclerotic disease, with 5 percent exhibiting severe disease.[6]

In autopsies performed at the University of Louisville in Kentucky on young, mostly male victims of trauma (average age twenty-six), coronary atherosclerosis was observed in 78 percent of the study group—with 21 percent showing narrowing of the coronary arteries by more than 50 percent, and 9 percent showing blockage of more than 75 percent.[7]

At this point, you may be thinking, what do all these scientific findings have to do with reversing *my* disease? The takeaway message that you should extract from the autopsy research is that your disease did not surface last year or last week but has been brewing in your arteries since you were a child. And, as you shall see, it took a lifetime of additional lifestyle factors to hasten its progression to the advanced stage that bred your critical cardiac event.

Multiple risk factors accelerate plaque buildup

Risk factors are traits people exhibit that increase their likelihood for contracting disease. Major risk factors for heart disease, such as high LDL or "bad" cholesterol, diabetes, high blood pressure, smoking, and obesity, have a detrimental effect on the lining of the innermost layer of the coronary arteries, the endothelium.[8]

One of the most important studies that proved beyond a

shadow of a doubt that these risk factors operate early in life in all Americans to propel atherosclerosis is the Bogalusa Heart Study. The longest and most detailed large-scale study of biracial children (black and white) in the world, the Bogalusa Heart Study began in 1972 in the town of Bogalusa, Louisiana, to determine the early course of heart disease and its association with established risk factors: lifestyle behaviors such as smoking, physical inactivity, and a high-fat, high-calorie diet. In an autopsy segment of the study, conducted at Tulane University Medical Center in New Orleans, researchers examined the coronary arteries of 204 young people between ages two and thirty-nine. (Most subjects had died from accidents.) The researchers found that 50 percent of the children age two to fifteen exhibited fatty streaks (the first visible sign of disease in the arteries), and 8 percent had full-blown plaque in their coronary arteries. The older group, age twenty-one to thirty-nine, had more advanced disease, with 85 percent having fatty streaks and 69 percent showing plaque in their coronary arteries.[9] Hence, the Bogalusa Heart Study has changed the way we think about heart disease, which was formerly considered an adult problem. The study proved that heart disease can start the day you are born and that poor lifestyle choices made in childhood can have deadly effects later in life.

Young Americans living dangerously: More research proves the point

Findings from the Pathobiological Determinants of Atherosclerosis in Youth (PDAY) study provide even more support for the notion that multiple risk factors accelerate the atherosclerotic process in young people. Scientists autopsied 2,876 young accident victims (age fifteen to thirty-four) and examined their coronary arteries for evidence of heart disease. Confirmation of atherosclerosis was found in an astounding 60 percent of subjects in the youngest group (age fifteen to nineteen), escalating to greater than 80 percent of men and 70 percent of women in the oldest group (age thirty to thirty-four).[10]

The PDAY study clarifies not only that atherosclerosis begins in youth but also that the risk factors for adult heart disease, if they appear at a young age, determine to a large degree the rate of progression of atherosclerotic plaque. Risk factors operating on young, vulnerable coronary arteries are the harbinger of future heart attacks, which will most likely appear at even younger ages in adulthood than currently observed.

CHILDHOOD OBESITY AND HEART DISEASE

The research is clear: Childhood obesity increases the risk of atherosclerosis and premature death in adulthood,[11] which is why the explosion of childhood obesity should be of great concern to all Americans. A recent *New York Times* article reported on research conducted at the University of Missouri–Kansas City School of Medicine.[12] The scientists examined the thickness of neck arteries of obese children and adolescents between ages six and nineteen. The children also exhibited high levels of LDL (or "plaque-building" cholesterol), triglycerides (another type of artery-clogging blood fat), high blood pressure, and low levels of HDL (or "good") cholesterol—all modifiable risk factors for CAD. Early warning signs of heart disease were clearly evident in the subjects. An ultrasound revealed that the subjects' arteries—and keep in mind that the subjects were all children and teenagers—resembled the "vascular age" of an average forty-five-year-old.

Further proof that the appearance of risk factors in children will increase the likelihood of a heart attack down the road comes from a Danish study that followed health statistics of more than 250,000 children into adulthood.[13] The authors found that the higher the childhood body weight, the greater the risk of heart disease in adulthood. A thirteen-year-old boy weighing about twenty-five pounds more than average, for example, would increase his risk of having a heart attack before age sixty by 33 percent—a graphic illustration of the harmful effects of childhood risk factors on future adult health.

PROTECT YOUR CHILDREN AS CHILDHOOD OBESITY THREATENS THEIR LIFE EXPECTANCY

Linking the current childhood obesity epidemic to future heart disease, a computer-generated forecast model predicts heart disease rates 5 percent to 16 percent higher than they are today—adding more than 100,000 cases by 2035. Scientists forecast that the disease-promoting effects of childhood obesity will threaten our nation's children such that they will live less healthy and possibly even *shorter lives than their parents.* For parents, this knowledge that heart disease begins in childhood and rapidly progresses to full-blown heart disease in adulthood should highlight the need for more aggressive action to control obesity in our children. Taking action now will help to stem the tide of heart disease sure to curtail the lives of future generations.

Sources: Kirsten Bibbins-Domingo et al., "Adolescent overweight and future adult coronary heart disease," *New England Journal of Medicine* 367, no. 23 (2007): 2371–2379; and S. Jay Olshansky et al., "A potential decline in life expectancy in the United States in the 21st century," *New England Journal of Medicine* 352, no. 11 (2005): 1138–1145.

A STRATEGY FOR YOUR AND YOUR DESCENDANTS' SURVIVAL IS IN YOUR HANDS

You are now fully aware of the tremendous importance of aggressively controlling heart disease risk factors in your children, who by virtue of their genes are at high risk for developing your disease in adulthood. So now, let's shift the focus back to you and take a look at the best strategy for preventing and reversing your disease.

As a heart attack survivor, you should make prevention of a second attack your top priority. Why? Having survived a heart attack, you are categorized as "high risk" for having another. According to the American Heart Association (AHA), one out of three women and one out of four men will die within the year of having their first heart attack, from either another attack or sudden cardiac arrest. Obviously, changes must be made to prevent that second cardiac event.

Unfortunately, medications alone can't reverse the atherosclerotic disease process. You need to make lifestyle changes, too—all of which are outlined in this book. The foods and the exercise prescribed in *Prevent a Second Heart Attack* fight off heart disease by targeting what has been referred to as the *trilogy of vulnerability,*[14] which are the three most vulnerable zones for high-risk cardiac patients: plaque, blood, and the heart muscle. As you will soon learn, when paired with the best modern medicine, a Mediterranean lifestyle plan can do three things:

1. Stabilize the high-risk, rupture-prone vulnerable plaque (the type responsible for most heart attacks) and reduce the likelihood that the plaque will rupture, which could result in another and potentially fatal heart attack.

2. Stabilize vulnerable blood—the composition of which is prone to form blood clots easily.

3. Stabilize a vulnerable heart muscle—the type that is prone to having arrhythmia or electrical instability.

But What About Drugs?

Although *Prevent a Second Heart Attack* specifically describes how lifestyle changes can lead to heart disease prevention and reversal, lifestyle is only part of the equation. All individuals who have experienced a heart attack can boost their survival odds by taking their physician-prescribed medication. (*Note:* The general information presented in this section regarding medications should not be used as medical advice. Please talk to your personal physician regarding which medications are right for you.)

FILL (AND TAKE) YOUR PRESCRIPTION MEDICATIONS!

A new study out of Canada analyzed drug adherence from 4,591 patients who had survived a heart attack. They found that only three out of four cardiac patients leaving the hospital filled all of their prescriptions. When compared to those people who filled all of their prescriptions:

• Patients who failed to fill any of their prescriptions had an 80 percent greater chance of dying in the year following their heart attack.

• Patients who filled only some of their prescriptions had a 40 percent increase in risk of death in the year following their heart attack.

Sources: Cynthia A. Jackevicius, Ping Li, and Jack V. Tu, "Prevalence, predictors, and outcomes of primary nonadherence after myocardial infarction," *Circulation* 117 (2008): 1028–1036; and Varda Shalev et al., "Continuation of statin treatment and all-cause mortality," *Archives of Internal Medicine* 169 (2009): 260–268.

According to the AHA's most recent guidelines for treating individuals with established heart disease, most patients would derive benefits from taking four types, or classes, of medications:

- **Cholesterol-lowering medications,** such as a statin drug like Lipitor
- **ACE (angiotensin-converting enzyme) inhibitors,** a medication that blocks a blood vessel constriction enzyme, such as Lotensin
- **Aspirin,** an anti-inflammatory drug that also lessens the ability of blood platelets to stick together and form a clot in the coronary arteries
- **Beta-blockers,** drugs that lessen the workload of the heart, such as Toprol[15]

Cholesterol targets: Down with the "bad," up with the"good"

Much controversy exists regarding the optimal level of cholesterol—both "good" HDL cholesterol and "bad" LDL cholesterol—for the prevention of heart disease. One thing is clear, though: Because you have had a previous heart attack and are thus considered high risk, you should aim for getting your LDL down to the lowest goal recommended, less than 70 mg/dL. (In fact, other scientists have stated that in people with diagnosed heart disease, a blood LDL level of *less than 40 mg/dL* is the number to strive for to completely halt progression of plaque buildup.[16]) This goal (less than 70 mg/dL) can be achieved by combining lifestyle (diet and exercise) with a low-dose statin medication.[17]

I suggest you follow the ten steps outlined in my previous book, *Cholesterol Down* (Three Rivers Press), to help you achieve an LDL value of less than 70 mg/dL and boost the cholesterol-lowering power of your prescription medication. Here are my ten daily LDL-cholesterol lowering steps in a nutshell:

CHOLESTEROL *AND* BLOOD PRESSURE DOWN = BEST PAYOFF FOR SLOWING ATHEROSCLEROSIS

A new study published in the *Journal of the American College of Cardiology* took the results of seven large clinical trials of patients with diagnosed CAD and rolled them all into one major recommendation: Get your LDL down to 70 mg/dL or less and your top blood pressure number (systolic pressure) to a normal value of 120 mm Hg or less and you will have the best results in halting plaque progression and promoting regression.

Source: Adnan K. Chhatriwalla et al., "Low levels of low-density lipoprotein cholesterol and blood pressure and progression of coronary atherosclerosis," *Journal of the American College of Cardiology* 53 (2009): 1110–1115.

---

1. Eat 1 cup of oatmeal every day (most therapeutic dose: 3 grams of beta-glucan fiber per day).

2. Eat a handful of almonds every day (most therapeutic dose: 1.5 ounces or approximately 30 almonds per day).

3. Eat 2 tablespoons of ground flaxseeds every day (3 grams of alpha-linolenic acid, or ALA).

4. Consume 3 grams (starting dose) to 10 grams (most therapeutic dose) of psyllium husk every day.

5. Eat ½ cup of legumes (beans, peas, or lentils) every day.

6. Eat 1 apple every day.

7. Consume 2–3 grams of phytosterols per day, preferably taken at three separate meals.

8. Eat 20–25 grams of soy protein every day.

9. Eat a clove of fresh garlic and take one Kyolic One Per Day Cardiovascular aged garlic extract supplement every day.

10. Walk for 30 minutes every day.

You know you need to cut down your "bad" cholesterol, but what about the "good" cholesterol, HDL? It's not enough protection to just get your LDL under control. You also need to raise your HDL cholesterol, because low HDL (defined as less than 40 mg/dL) can greatly increase your risk for another heart attack. Individuals with really low HDL (<35 mg/dL) have eight times the risk of heart disease compared to those with a high HDL (>65 mg/dL).[18] If all of these numbers seem confusing, I'll make it easy for you: To reach your "ideal" cholesterol levels, *keep "good" HDL above 60 and "bad" LDL below 70.*

The best way to bump up your good cholesterol value safely is to lose weight (if you are overweight), stop smoking, and follow the diet and exercise advice outlined in this book. As far as medications to raise HDL, there are not as many choices as there are for lowering LDL. Statins (cholesterol-lowering medications such as Lipitor) and drugs called fibrates (such as Lopid) both increase HDL to varying degrees. However, they also have side effects, so they must be taken under a doctor's close medical supervision.

NIACIN: AN UNDERUSED STRATEGY FOR BUMPING UP YOUR HDL

What are the best lifestyle steps to take to get your HDL to climb to new heights? As you will soon learn, moderate alcohol consumption (drinking your daily red wine prescription) is associated with the largest incremental increase in HDL, but getting in your daily exercise will also make a measurable difference. If you are overweight, losing weight will increase HDL, as will following the Mediterranean-style eating strategy outlined in these pages. Because cigarette smoking lowers HDL, quitting smoking will also boost your good cholesterol level.

You should also consider taking niacin, the B vitamin available over the counter or as a prescription drug—proven to possess the greatest capacity to increase your blood level of HDL compared to other drugs. The immediate-release form of niacin, taken at a high dose of 3 grams per day, raises HDL by about 30 percent. The film-coated, slow-release form of niacin, marketed as the prescription drug Niaspan (Abbott Laboratories), increases HDL by 10 to 30 percent. Combining niacin with your statin medication can shrink artery plaque, according to a new study out of the United Kingdom. Two grams a day of Niaspan, on top of statins, resulted in a 1.64-mm^2 reduction in plaque in the neck arteries of subjects with coronary artery disease. What's more, after twelve months, the niacin group increased HDL by 23 percent and decreased LDL by 19 percent. Another recent study examined the plaque thickness of the neck arteries of 208 patients with heart disease on statin medication taking either Niaspan (up to 2 grams a day) or Zetia (Merck/Schering-Plough) (10 milligrams per day) for 12 months. Niacin clearly had a superior effect on the artery wall, reducing plaque by about 2 percent compared to an increase in plaque progression with Zetia.

With more than thirty years of research supporting the safety and effectiveness of the old standby drug niacin, you and your doctor should discuss adding this vitamin as a second agent on top of your statin to boost your fight against plaque. The problem with niacin is its potential side effects, which include flushing, itching, and gastrointestinal upset. The extended-release form reduces these unpleasant side effects. Taking aspirin one hour before ingesting niacin as well as avoiding spicy foods, saturated fat, and hot liquids for three hours before taking it also helps quell the flushing. Because niacin has the potential to cause adverse side effects, I recommend you take it only under your doctor's supervision.

Sources: Peter P. Toth, "When high is low: Raising low levels of high-density lipoprotein cholesterol," *Current Cardiology Reports* 10 (2008): 488–496; Justin M. S. Lee et al., "Effects of high-dose modified-release nicotinic acid on atherosclerosis and vascular function," *Journal of the American College of Cardiology* 54, no. 19 (2009): 1787–1794; and Allen J. Taylor et al., "Extended-release niacin or ezetimibe and carotid intima-media thickness," *New England Journal of Medicine* (2009): doi: 10.1056/NEJMoa0907569.

THE CHILD IS FATHER OF THE MAN

In this chapter, you have learned that your disease has been developing within you since you were a child. You understand that a lifetime of exposure to a Western diet of artery-clogging foods coupled with inactivity has fueled your disease process until eventually it surfaced and you had a wake-up call—the event that changed your life. Obviously, as a heart attack survivor, you realize that you were predisposed to the disease. Take this knowledge and apply it to your children, as there's a very good chance that your children and your children's children will be in the same boat as you—or perhaps may not have the good fortune to survive. Be sure to instill the heart-healthy eating and exercise habits outlined in these pages early on in your children's lives, for as William Wordsworth so eloquently wrote in his classic poem "The Rainbow," "The child is father of the man." What we are when we are young gives shape to the adult that we become and will remain with us forever.

You have also learned that all is not hopeless, that you can take control of your disease, halt its progression, and even promote its regression by taking aggressive action to tame your risk factors and target your "trilogy of vulnerability" by taking your medication and rearranging your cholesterol numbers, all in combination with a new diet and exercise lifestyle plan. But before we discuss the exact makeup of the Prevent a Second Heart Attack Mediterranean lifestyle to pair with your medication as the optimal prescription for cardioprotection, I ask that you join me and take a trip deep down into your coronary arteries. In this next chapter you will learn the science behind the process of atherosclerosis— so you can see from a cellular point of view just how you got heart disease in the first place and exactly how and why your new lifestyle will beat this disease.

Atherosclerosis: A Story of Inflammation, Plaque, and Death of a Heart Muscle

An investment in knowledge always pays the best interest.

—Benjamin Franklin, American inventor and statesman (1706–1790)

NEW VIEW OF HEART DISEASE

As you have learned, heart disease does not happen overnight. It is a long, slow process that often begins in childhood and can take decades to evolve. Suddenly, often without any warning, a series of events occurs in one of the clogged arteries that feeds the heart, and a potentially fatal heart attack ensues.

No longer is heart disease considered simply a "plumbing problem." Doctors once thought a heart attack was the result of a "pipe" clogging up—like your sink pipe clogging up with a glob of hair, blocking water flow, and backing up. It was believed that fatty deposits of cholesterol, cells, calcium, muscle tissue, and other cellular debris (plaque) build up on the artery walls and expand so large that they choke off blood flow, and *bam*—there is your heart attack. Scientists now know that these kinds of plaque deposits, the type that almost totally clog your arteries—expanding to the point of nearly preventing blood from reaching the heart—are *not* the most dangerous. In fact, most heart attacks occur when smaller, less obtrusive but highly inflamed plaque bursts open. This event triggers the formation of a large, totally obstructive blood clot in an artery. It is this clot (or thrombus) *and not the plaque* that blocks the flow of blood, thus causing cellular death of some of your heart muscle downstream of the blockage (heart attack).

You have been there. You have survived a heart attack, and your life has changed forever. Now your focus is on *secondary prevention,* a medical term that represents strategies used to prevent the recurrence of atherosclerotic heart disease or a second heart attack. But to appreciate the basis for secondary prevention therapy, you must first understand the disease process itself.

I encourage you to read this chapter closely and take a guided tour deep within your arteries and see for yourself, up close and personal, how perfectly healthy arteries develop into dysfunctional, diseased arteries. Learn about how atherosclerosis—the treacherous disease of the arteries—begins, how it progresses, and how it almost killed you. In so doing, you will arm yourself with knowledge you can use to better comprehend the rationale for the heart attack prevention and reversal strategies set forth in this book.

ATHEROSCLEROSIS: THE UNDERLYING CAUSE OF HEART DISEASE

A heart attack is almost always due to atherosclerotic disease of the coronary arteries. The term *atherosclerosis* (ATH-er-o-skleh-RO-sis), which is derived from the Greek word for "gruel" or "hardening," is the buildup of plaque—semihard material consisting of cholesterol and other substances—that accumulates in the inner lining of the artery wall. Plaque is also called a *lesion* in the medical world—an abnormal growth in the artery wall that is the result of disease. Atherosclerotic plaques, in various stages of evolution, are widely dispersed within the coronary arteries of patients with CAD. Hence, heart disease is actually not a disease of the *entire heart* but instead is a malfunction of select areas within the heart's own blood supply network, or more precisely, within the layer of microscopic cells—indistinguishable to the human eye—that line the inner wall of the heart's blood vessels, or the *endothelium*.

You are not alone. Atherosclerosis—the root cause of heart disease—is so common that it is predicted to be the principal cause of death for all human beings on the planet by the year 2020.[1] You are aware that atherosclerosis starts at a young age, silently and relentlessly progressing over decades. What is most disturbing, though, is that the progression of atherosclerosis is not linear with time, nor predictable. In fact, dangerous "vulnerable" plaque can appear in coronary arteries that were normal on an angiogram just months earlier.[2]

Plaque buildup is a multistage process. It begins with the appearance of fatty patches or streaks (more about those later) within the arterial wall and can progress, like a cancer, with the plaque growing and spreading within the coronary arteries like tumors. Eventually, some of the fatty patches or streaks may develop into "vulnerable plaque"—which although it is asymptomatic (i.e., doesn't create any symptoms), is actually the most precarious type of plaque because it is so rupture prone. Most plaque forms at the *branch points,* or bends in the arterial tree, of the medium- and large-sized arteries that feed the heart (Figure 2.1). (The major arteries in your heart are quite small, about the size of spaghetti strands.) So common and deadly is the occurrence of atherosclerosis in one particular coronary artery, the left anterior descending artery, that this artery is sometimes referred to as "the widow-maker."

Danger Zones: Where Plaque Forms

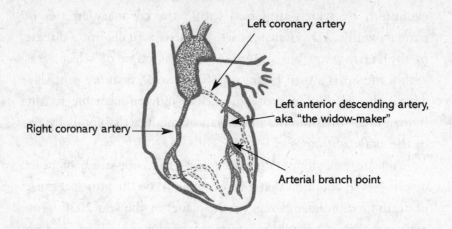

Left coronary artery

Left anterior descending artery, aka "the widow-maker"

Right coronary artery

Arterial branch point

Figure 2.1 Plaque, and especially "vulnerable plaque," the most dangerous type, tends to form at the arterial branch points—the splits in the arteries that feed the heart.

Inside a healthy artery

The heart is a muscle, about the size of your fist, and functions as a pump to generate the pressure needed to get the blood flowing along the miles of arteries in the body. The heart has its own special collection of arteries, the coronary arteries, which carry blood and nutrients such as oxygen to the heart muscle cells.

Arteries are circular in cross section and contain three distinct layers: the innermost layer, the intima; the middle or muscular layer, the media; and the external layer, the adventitia. Figure 2.2 shows the anatomy of a healthy artery.

Endothelial lining

The endothelial lining is composed of endothelial cells that form the first thin layer on the interior of the arteries. The endothelium resembles a single sheet of flattened pancakes all attached to one another, with microscopic junctions between each "pancake," or endothelial lining cell. This innermost layer, adjacent to the flow of

Inside a Healthy Coronary Artery

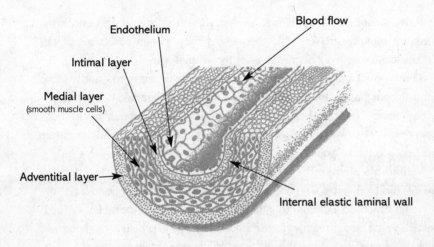

Figure 2.2 A cross-sectional view of a normal, healthy coronary artery. Arteries consist of three layers: the intima, the media, and the adventitia. Coating the innermost layer, the intima, is a layer of smooth, flat endothelial cells collectively referred to as the endothelium.

blood, is normally silky smooth and resists cells from the bloodstream adhering to it. This is Mother Nature's way of preventing abnormal blood clotting. The endothelial cells serve as a barrier between the blood and the inner layer of the arterial pipes, the intima. A healthy endothelium has three notable characteristics: (1) It produces chemicals that keep the arteries relaxed and dilated; (2) it has tight junctions between the cells that block entry of anything abnormal from the blood into the intimal layer; and (3) it does not generate chemicals or molecules that let immune system cells or platelets (blood-clotting cells) stick to its surface. *Endothelial lining cells are extremely important in the process of atherosclerosis, as their dysfunction is the root cause of heart disease.*

Intimal layer

The first layer of the artery, the intimal layer, consists of a mostly cell-free spongy substance. A few muscle cells are scattered within

PLAQUE 101

• **Fatty streaks.** The first hint of disease within the coronary arteries is the appearance of fatty streaks—thin yellow lines that contain collections of fat-filled cells located within the inner layer of the arterial wall.

• **Transitional plaque.** Over time, some fatty streaks may grow and develop into transitional plaque, the precursor for the more advanced and dangerous vulnerable plaque. Transitional plaque is located deeper within the intima and has smooth muscle cell involvement, which contributes to the stringy or fibrous nature of the newly formed plaque.

• **Vulnerable plaque.** This advanced type of plaque is of greatest concern because it is this type that is the underlying cause of heart attacks. Fueled by inflammation and continued exposure to irritating risk factors (i.e., excess LDL or "bad" cholesterol in the bloodstream, cigarette smoke, high blood pressure, or abnormally high blood sugar levels), vulnerable plaque falls into one of two categories:

  • **Hard nonrupture-prone plaque.** This hard, thick, calcium-filled *stenotic* plaque clogs up the arteries. It grows inward, restricting blood supply, hence causing the chest pain or discomfort felt during periods of *angina* (the medical term for these symptoms). Nonrupture-prone plaque is responsible for roughly 30 percent of deaths from heart attacks.

  • **Soft rupture-prone plaque.** This volatile plaque is softer, smaller, and less stable than stenotic plaque and *is responsible for approximately 70 percent of deaths from heart attacks;* thus it is considered the most high-risk type. Most lethal heart attacks stem from these cholesterol- and pus-filled, highly inflamed pimple-like growths. Many people with heart disease have not one but *multiple vulnerable plaques* permeating their entire coronary arterial tree.

Sources: Morteza Naghavi et al., "From vulnerable plaque to vulnerable patient: A call for new definitions and risk assessment strategies: Part I," *Circulation* 108 (2003): 1664–1672; Luigi Giusto Spagnoli et al., "Role of inflammation in atherosclerosis," *Journal of Nuclear Medicine* 48 (2007): 1800–1815; and Renu Virmani et al., "Pathology of unstable plaque," *Progress in Cardiovascular Diseases* 44 (2002): 349–356.

the intima to produce the stabilizing components, or framework, of the intimal layer. A healthy artery also contains an intact wavy line called the internal elastic laminal wall, located on the outer portion of the intimal layer; this wall acts as an additional barrier to keep smooth muscle cell neighbors sequestered where they belong, in their own medial layer. *In atherosclerosis, most of the plaque formation takes place in the intimal layer.*

Medial layer

The media, or middle layer of the artery, is basically a circular ring of muscle tissue. The media contains masses of tightly packed muscle cells and some elastic connective tissue. Healthy arteries contain a complete layer of these muscle cells, *smooth muscle cells,* cordoned off in their own space, the medial layer. *In atherosclerosis, the smooth muscle cells play a destructive role by exhibiting highly abnormal behavior.*

Adventitial layer

The outer layer of the artery, the adventitia, consists mainly of elastic tissue that is capable of expanding, helping the blood vessel to manage the high pressures that result from turbulent blood flow. With each beat of the heart, the blood vessels swell, and the elastic nature of the outer arterial wall allows for this expansion. The muscular tissue (smooth muscle cells) then contracts and squeezes the blood along the arterial highways, allowing the blood to circulate to cells throughout the body. *The adventitial layer does not play much of a role in plaque buildup other than its involvement in inflammation.*

HOW ATHEROSCLEROSIS DEVELOPS

Accumulation of cholesterol fuels inflammation

Atherosclerosis involves an abnormal uptake of low-density lipoprotein (LDL), or "bad" cholesterol, into the arterial wall. Thus LDL cholesterol is a key building block of plaque. It is important to understand that *atherosclerosis is primarily a disease of cholesterol deposition.* This is why driving down your circulating level of LDL cholesterol is crucial for preventing another heart attack. Less

> ## INFLAMMATION: FRIEND AND FOE
>
> Inflammation is a normal, necessary bodily function and occurs when your system is fighting off an infection or healing an injury. If you get a splinter in your finger, you will notice signs of inflammation—redness, swelling, heat, and pain at the site of the injury. This is an *acute* inflammatory reaction, one that dissipates over time. In the case of atherosclerosis in the coronary arteries, the inflammatory reaction—a localized response to *ongoing* arterial injury—is *chronic,* and ultimately a harmful one. *This kind of inflammation is a bodily response gone haywire, a healing response by the body that promotes increased plaque formation and fuels the atherosclerotic disease process.* To halt and reverse your disease, the arterial inflammation must be extinguished and the arterial milieu converted to a healthy, less agitated state.

LDL in the bloodstream attacks the root cause of the disease— *inflammation.* Plus, maintaining a very low blood level of LDL will prevent further deposition of cholesterol into the plaque, halting progression of plaque and thereby stabilizing the most precarious type of fatty cholesterol-filled vulnerable plaque that already exists in your arteries.

Once LDL has pierced the artery wall, it triggers the *activation* of the endothelial lining cells. Activation is a maladaptive and harmful series of biological inflammatory responses—a vicious cycle occurring within the endothelial cells that promotes further plaque deposition.[3] Upon activation, the endothelial cells are transformed from healthy to dysfunctional as they try to counteract the plaque (perceived as a threat to the body, which responds via heightened inflammation). The most dangerous forms of atherosclerotic plaques—those responsible for the greatest number of deaths from a heart attack—are those that display the most chronic inflammation.[4]

Fatty streaks—first sign of disease. The inflammatory atherosclerotic process begins with the formation of a *fatty streak*. Fatty streaks are thin yellow cholesterol deposits embedded in the arterial wall. Fatty streaks are frequently observed in the coronary arteries of children and adolescents and are even commonly seen in the ar-

DO YOU KNOW YOUR CHOLESTEROL PARTICLE SIZE?

When it comes to the size of your cholesterol particles (both "good" HDL and "bad" LDL), remember . . . bigger is better! Small, heavy LDL particles are much more dangerous than larger, fluffier ones. Individuals with diagnosed heart disease generally exhibit a large number of the small, heavy type of LDL. These particles can more easily squeeze through the tiny junctions that lie between each of the endothelial cells blanketing the inner arterial wall. The smaller particles are also more susceptible to oxidation and remain in the bloodstream longer than the larger types, so they are considered highly *atherogenic,* meaning they are willing participants in atherosclerosis. Bigger and more plentiful HDL particles are also the healthier version, so a low number of small HDL particles is a common characteristic of patients with heart disease. Some of the foods and exercise prescribed in *Prevent a Second Heart Attack* can help rearrange your LDL and HDL particle size and number. For example, you can reduce your LDL number as well as morph the composition from the small, dangerous type to the healthier, larger, lighter version and bump up the number and size of your HDLs too. Ask your doctor about getting a new series of blood cholesterol tests from the Berkeley HeartLab. The results will help you and your doctor track the positive changes in size and number of your cholesterol particles that will result from your diet and lifestyle changes.

teries of infants.[5] (This is not a natural process and appears in an infant's coronary arteries only when there is high circulating maternal cholesterol—all too common in Western societies.) Fatty streak formation begins when high amounts of blood-borne LDL cholesterol particles are absorbed into the intima and ravaged by chemicals (oxidized or *modified*). Once the LDL has been irreparably altered, it is perceived by the body as a foreign invader and your immune system takes action. Soon, two types of white blood cells arrive from the bloodstream and enter into the intimal layer. Within the intima, the modified cholesterol-filled LDL is then engulfed by one type of immune system cell in particular, the macrophage scavenger cell. The scavenger cell ingests the cholesterol, forming *foam*

Fatty Streak Formation

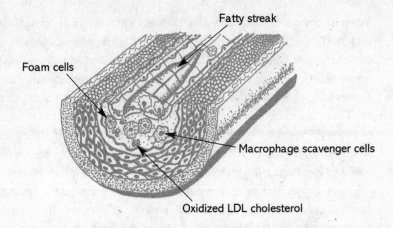

Figure 2.3. Cross-section of a fatty streak located within the intima of the coronary artery wall. The formation of fatty streaks is driven by an inflammatory response to injury. LDL enters the intima and is oxidized and engulfed by macrophages, forming foam cells, the type of cell that characterizes the atherosclerotic process.

cells (Figure 2.3), so named for the cells' bubbly, fat-filled appearance. Foam cells are one of the earliest markers of disease and are the hallmark of the atherosclerotic process.[6]

Fatty streak formation is asymptomatic and can even be harmless if it disappears with time.[7] In many cases, however, fatty streaks are the precursor to a more worrisome form of abnormal arterial growth called *transitional plaque*. Several factors accelerate the transformation of the fatty streak into the first real stage of actual plaque formation, including the following:

- High concentrations of LDL in the blood, especially the small type highly susceptible to oxidation
- Fewer antioxidants in the bloodstream
- A genetic predisposition to LDL uptake in the arterial wall[8]

When fatty streaks become dangerous. Over time and with continued exposure to injurious elements (such as high blood pressure, high cholesterol, or cigarette smoke), some of the plaque continues to grow within the artery wall, progressing from the innocuous fatty streak to the more dangerous forms. Mature plaque buildup results from the interaction of different types of cells inside the inner arterial wall that intermingle together over time. Four types of cells in particular play leading roles in the atherosclerotic process: (1) endothelial cells (arterial "lining" cells), (2) white blood cells (immune system cells), (3) macrophage scavenger cells, and (4) smooth muscle cells (specialized muscle cells). Let's look at how each of these four types of cells perpetuates inflammation, the fuel for the fire that propagates the disease process of atherosclerosis.

DISEASED ENDOTHELIUM BECOMES DYSFUNCTIONAL

A healthy endothelium releases chemicals that cause the blood vessel to either contract or relax depending on whatever the situation calls for. A diseased or "dysfunctional" endothelium generates an abnormal amount of the chemicals that enhance *constriction* of the artery and blood clotting. *A dysfunctional endothelium is a predictor of future cardiac events and greatly increases your risk of a second heart attack.* As you will learn, steps in the Prevent a Second Heart Attack plan can boost the body's production of nitric oxide, the chemical that promotes the *relaxation* of the artery, as well as thins the blood, helping to promote a healthier endothelium.

Sources: Yiannis S. Chatzizisis et al., "Role of endothelial shear stress in the natural history of coronary atherosclerosis and vascular remodeling," *Journal of the American College of Cardiology* 49, no. 25 (2007): 2379–2393; and Joseph Yeboah et al., "Brachial flow-mediated dilation predicts incident cardiovascular events in older adults: The Cardiovascular Health Study," *Circulation* 115 (2007): 2390–2397.

Role of endothelial lining cells. Sensing a foreign invader (modified or oxidized LDL) within the intima, activated endothelial cells respond to the perceived invasion by sending out chemical distress signals into the blood. Activated endothelial cells also sprout Velcro-like *adhesion molecules* from their surface. Adhesion molecules make the artery wall sticky, enabling the immune system's white blood cells to attach to the endothelium. A healthy endothelium has a smooth surface that does not allow cells to stick to it, in order to prevent the clotting of blood platelets along its surface.[9] A diseased endothelium, however, is abnormally sticky; hence it allows white blood cells to adhere to its surface. To add to the danger, eventually the highly damaged endothelium also attracts harmful blood platelets, the tiny blood cell fragments that cause life-threatening clots.

Role of white blood cells. When they receive the message from endothelial cells, two types of white blood cells—monocytes and T lymphocytes (a.k.a. T cells)—that reside in the bloodstream are called to the battlefield (activated endothelium) to help fight off the enemy. The monocytes and T cells, both immune system cells, are the true culprits in fueling inflammation and promoting the growth of atherosclerotic plaque. The white blood cells stick to the inner wall of the artery. The cells adhere to Velcro-like adhesion molecules protruding from the cells of the endothelium. The immune cells then steamroll along the façade until they reach an abnormally widened crevice separating the irritated endothelial cells. At this point, they squeeze into the gaps between the endothelial cell walls, infiltrating the inner layer of the coronary artery, the intima. Once inside, the former blood-borne white blood cells now become permanent residents, perpetuating a long-lasting inflammatory reaction.

Although we normally think of white blood cells as a "healthy" part of the immune system's defenses, when they enter the inner wall of an artery, they fuel a dangerous and long-lasting inflammatory reaction. As you know, this "fire within" promotes the growth of atherosclerotic plaque. When monocytes, which are naturally blood-borne, become permanent residents of the arterial wall—that is to say, they leave the blood and install themselves in the intima—they mature into *macrophages,* from the Greek word for "big eaters." Read on to learn why this type of immune system cell was so aptly named.

Role of macrophages. Macrophages (which begin their lives as blood-borne white blood cells) are the key players in the body's immune response to foreign invaders such as bacteria and other infectious microorganisms. Within the intima, however, the macrophages are also known as *scavenger cells* because they have matured into large cells that grow *scavenger receptors* on their surface. This means that the macrophages hone in on the modified LDL and, using their scavenger receptors, feast on the fat-filled LDL uncontrollably. The scavenger receptors are trained to seek out and ingest only LDL that has been chemically modified or *oxidized*. In turn, the macrophages become engorged with cholesterol, bursting with fat. The macrophages have now been transformed into cholesterol-rich foam cells, all bubbly in composition. *If you could depress the uptake of cholesterol by macrophages, fewer foam cells would form and you could delay or reverse the progression of atherosclerosis.*

The macrophages continue to replicate, and foam cells begin to fuse together. Thus, large colonies of fat-filled foam cells are formed; *the cholesterol-rich foam cell colonies form the pools of fat characterizing vulnerable atherosclerotic plaque.* The overloaded mass of foam cells begins to die, and their cache of fat is unloaded and congeals with other smaller pools of fat, all located deep within the intima. This collusion of dead and decomposing macrophage foam cells forms little lakes of mostly cholesterol and dead foam cell remnants, giving the intima a Swiss cheese–like appearance. Eventually theses small fat pools coalesce into one large lake, forming the unstable plaque's *fatty core*[10] (Figure 2.4).

Role of smooth muscle cells. Smooth muscle cells also play a large role in the progression of plaque. In a healthy artery, smooth muscle

Four Cells (and Cholesterol) Contribute to Advanced Plaque Formation

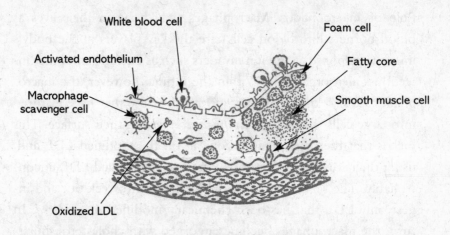

Figure 2.4. Four types of cells are involved in vulnerable plaque formation: activated endothelial cells, white blood cells (monocytes and T cells), macrophage scavenger cells, and smooth muscle cells (which are explained in the text). LDL cholesterol accumulates in the intimal layer of the artery and becomes oxidized. It is then ingested by macrophage scavenger cells and transformed into foam cells. Smooth muscle cells migrate into the intimal layer, contributing to plaque buildup. Chemicals are continuously secreted from various cells, perpetuating inflammation.

cells remain sequestered within their own layer—the media—for life. In diseased arteries, smooth muscle cells began to emigrate en masse from the medial layer by puncturing through and fragmenting a dividing wall that normally separates the middle layer from the inner arterial layer (the *internal elastic lamina*). Smooth muscle cells can also take up oxidized LDL, resulting in an additional source of plaque-building foam cells. In time, large numbers of smooth muscle cells migrate into the intima, where they both replicate and produce a more stable framework, thereby elaborating the density of the ever-growing plaque as well as increasing the growing plaque's role as a source of inflammation. While they are inside the inner layer, smooth muscle cells are stimulated to produce collagen and thus create a more definitive growth within the artery wall.

Note that the evolution of fatty streaks to more advanced plaque relies greatly on the unnatural involvement of smooth muscle cells.[11]

The following is a summary of early events leading to plaque formation:

1. LDL uptake, oxidation, and retention within the endothelium trigger a cascade of inflammation, resulting in expression of adhesion molecules along the endothelial surface.

2. Two types of white blood cells (monocytes and T lymphocytes) stick to the endothelium, roll along the surface, and pierce the endothelial layer.

3. Once inside, monocytes transform into macrophage scavengers (warped white blood cells) that actively seek out and consume oxidized LDL, forming foam cells, visible to the human eye as fatty streaks.

4. Progression of the disease occurs when a large lake of fat takes shape, smooth muscle cells migrate to the newly formed mass and proliferate, and the concentration of additional inflammatory cells and chemicals escalates.

THE ADVANCED PHASES OF ATHEROSCLEROSIS

In a process that may take months or decades, the most dangerous types of plaque form in the coronary arteries. This occurs when macrophages, foam cells, and T cells, in their efforts to fight modified LDL, continue to release inflammatory chemicals over time that stimulate a response from the endothelial cells to sprout more adhesion molecules. This response, in turn, amplifies the recruitment of more white blood cells and perpetuates the inflammatory response and the call for reinforcements. The migration of monocytes into the intimal layer is increased, more macrophages form, and the process intensifies. Intimal cells exude growth chemicals, stimulating enlargement of the lesion within the intima. Thus, the production of the weblike matrix that constitutes plaque is accelerated, and the nascent plaque may evolve into full-blown vulnerable types of plaque—the most worrisome kind, a result of chronic arterial damage from excess LDL cholesterol and inflammation.[12] There are two types of advanced and dangerous vulnerable plaque: hard, stable, nonrupture-prone plaque and soft, unstable, rupture-prone plaque.

Hard, stable, nonrupture-prone plaque

Years of plaque growth within the coronary arteries characteristic of advanced coronary artery disease often results in a hardened mass of calcified plaque and scar tissue that tends to protrude inward, such that it encroaches into the lumen, the cavity where the blood flows (Figure 2.5). Over time this fibrous plaque can impinge on the inner diameter, even occasionally progressing to a full occlusion of blood flow (complete clogging of the artery). This

Stable Versus Unstable Vulnerable Plaque

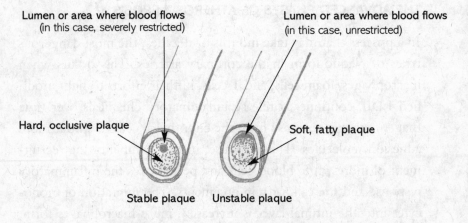

Lumen or area where blood flows (in this case, severely restricted)

Lumen or area where blood flows (in this case, unrestricted)

Hard, occlusive plaque

Soft, fatty plaque

Stable plaque   Unstable plaque

Figure 2.5. The more stable type of calcium-filled occlusive plaque grows inward, restricting blood flow. The more volatile, soft, vulnerable plaque grows differently. The artery shown on the right is highly inflamed and bulges outward, with a large, soft, fatty mass located within the intima.

type of growth characterizes the *stenotic,* nonrupture-prone vulnerable plaque that causes chest pain (angina), due to restricted blood flow to the heart muscle downstream. When nitroglycerin, a potent blood vessel dilator, is placed under the tongue, it is quickly absorbed and dilates the clogged artery, increasing blood flow and easing pain.

The coronary artery adapts to stenotic plaque by stretching outward and can reach almost twice its normal size to compensate for reduction in blood flow. Stenotic plaque can be deadly. In a small percentage of cases, this type of plaque—the kind that is not inflamed but can grow to fully obstruct the artery—can cause complications. If it *erodes,* or develops calcium deposits in or near the scablike covering that forms to separate the plaque from the blood, a clot can grow, leading to a heart attack.

Soft, unstable, rupture-prone plaque

Unlike stable plaque, soft and inflamed rupture-prone plaque tends to grow stealthily inside the arterial wall, where the ballooning plaque is pushed outward and away from the flow of blood. The outward bulge preserves much of the inner diameter of the lumen, the

---

ANGIOGRAMS DO NOT TELL THE WHOLE STORY ABOUT PLAQUE

As noted previously, it is not the size of the plaque but its stability that correlates with having a heart attack. In fact, the smaller, yet highly inflamed, ubiquitous plaque that burrows and hides deep within the arterial wall is most prone to rupturing and triggering a heart attack. Because this high-risk, unstable, rupture-prone type of vulnerable plaque grows outward, it is frequently *not detectable angiographically,* whereas the more stable, stenotic plaque is clearly evident. Therefore, although angiograms are valuable clinical tools for diagnosing heart disease, they are not a valid means of detecting the most precarious form of plaque, the unstable, rupture-prone vulnerable plaque, because they are simply not clearly visible on an angiogram.

Source: V. Stephen Monroe, Leonard D. Parilak, and Richard A. Kerensky, "Angiographic patterns and the natural history of the vulnerable plaque," *Progress in Cardiovascular Diseases* 44, no. 5 (2002): 339–347.

diameter of the artery where the blood flows. This type of plaque does not result in symptoms of angina, as blood flow is rarely compromised to any great degree. This adaptive response to plaque was once thought to be a "positive" occurrence because it did not clog up the artery—the old view of what causes a heart attack—by preserving the diameter of the lumen. Now we know that this type of growth is certainly not "positive," because this growth pattern weakens the plaque and is characteristic of the more deadly type in which inflammation is deeply involved—the high-risk, rupture-prone vulnerable plaque (Figure 2.5).

Autopsy studies: Soft, vulnerable plaque is responsible for most heart attacks

Detailed autopsy studies have revealed distinct characteristics of the type of plaque that predisposes individuals to an acute coronary event. These studies have determined that most heart attacks stem from events involving the small yet high-risk, rupture-prone plaque. One of the most defining characteristics of this killer plaque is the fat-filled core, often called the *necrotic core,* named for the lake of dead, fatty foam cells and macrophages that lie inside. Additional constituents of the fluid lake include cholesterol, which consists of different types of fluid cholesterol as well as pieces of crystallized cholesterol; oxidized LDL cholesterol; and cellular debris.[13] Autopsies of people who died of coronary atherosclerosis have shown *a much higher prevalence of soft plaques that contain a fat-rich core* compared to the more advanced, hard types of calcified stenotic plaques.[14] This is because the larger fatty core makes this plaque more unstable.

Let's take a closer look at the role of the vulnerable plaque's fibrous "cap." As the pool of fat located deep within the intima continues to expand across the intimal layer, it moves toward the endothelium and the river of blood. Smooth muscle cells also migrate toward the lumen, where the blood flows. Over the top of the vul-

Formation of Vulnerable Rupture-Prone Plaque

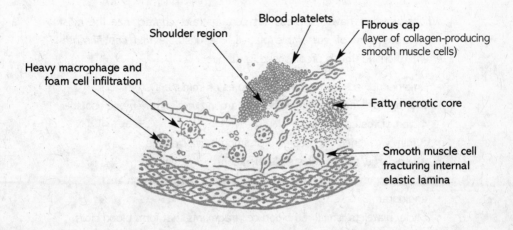

Figure 2.6. Note the large fat pool, fractured internal elastic lamina, macrophage scavenger cells, foam cells, smooth muscle cell involvement forming a thick fibrous cap, and large mass of blood platelets sticking to the activated endothelium.

nerable plaque grows a layer of connective tissue (produced by the smooth muscle cells), aptly named the fibrous *cap*, which cordons off the fatty core of the plaque from the bloodstream. The cap resembles a scab on a wound and sequesters the mature atherosclerotic mountain of fat-filled plaque from the river of blood flowing through the artery (Figure 2.6).

Thinning of the cap: Prelude to disaster. Normally, smooth muscle cells residing in the plaque cap produce plenty of collagen, which keeps the cap strong and prevents the contents within the volcano-like plaque from erupting. This scenario results in a strong and thick cap, a secure form of plaque that is less likely to rupture. (Note that the stable type of stenotic plaque is characterized by a thick, rupture-proof fibrous cap.)

In the later stages of vulnerable, rupture-prone plaque development, however, continued inflammation results in a thinning of the "cap" of cells that covers the plaque separating it from the

CHARACTERISTICS OF KILLER PLAQUE

Autopsy studies have revealed that certain traits characterize the most treacherous form of vulnerable plaque, the unstable *thin cap fibroatheroma,* the kind that is predisposed to rupture:

- Smoldering, active inflammation (scores of immune system cells: macrophages and T cells), especially around the fracture-prone shoulder region of the cap
- A thin, weakened cap depleted of smooth muscle cells
- A very large, fatty, cholesterol-laden core
- Outward growth within the arterial wall, not detectable on an angiogram
- Sticky platelets (small red blood cell fragments that form blood clots) ready and able to quickly clot and aggregate on the endothelial surface

bloodstream. (A thin fibrous cap overlying a highly inflamed, macrophage-rich core is a hallmark of the lethal *thin cap fibroatheroma,* the most dangerous kind of plaque that causes most heart attacks.) Malfunctioning immune system cells (macrophages and T cells) join together and launch a double assault on the all-important collagen-producing smooth muscle cells of the fibrous cap. The consequences of these actions are devastating:

1. Smooth muscle cells stop making collagen for cap and plaque maintenance, and hence the cap structure weakens.

2. Immune system cells infiltrate the cap, releasing toxic chemicals (free radicals and enzymes) that degrade the components that keep the fibrous cap strong.[15]

3. Smooth muscle cells die, leading to an increase in cellular debris and a lack of smooth muscle cell support.

4. *The fibrous cap becomes irreparably weakened and frail;* in turn, the plaque becomes highly unstable and vulnerable to rupture, resulting in the formation of a thin cap fibroatheroma.

Vulnerable plaque rupture. Vulnerable rupture-prone plaque can lead to death under certain conditions. The precarious series of events generally occurs as follows: Eventually, the sizable fatty inner core of the plaque—teeming with inflammatory pus cells (macrophages)—combined with the weakened cap becomes dangerously susceptible to the great mechanical force of circulating blood. When the stress becomes too much for the thin, weakened cap, as when an additional aggravating factor such as an early morning spike in blood pressure occurs, the plaque bursts.

The clot that seals your fate. Once the fibrous cap has fractured, volumes of flowing blood come in contact with the contents of the inner core—the cholesterol, cholesterol crystals, calcium, and cell debris. The inflammatory cells within the plaque send out signals

---

WHAT CAUSES MASSIVE PLAQUE RUPTURE?

Vulnerable plaque can rupture without any apparent stimulus. **Certain key external factors** increase the likelihood of the massive rupture of a weakened, vulnerable thin cap plaque:

- **Time of day** (Most heart attacks occur in the early morning, possibly related to an increase in blood pressure from rising out of bed.)
- **Time of year** (Heart attacks occur more often in the stressful winter months, especially during the first week of daylight saving time, when there is a spike in heart attacks of between 6 percent and 10 percent.)
- **Extreme physical exertion** (For example, shoveling snow puts much stress on the heart due to the sole use of upper-body muscles.)
- **Anger** (as experienced in a violent quarrel)
- **Severe emotional stress** (as experienced in a natural disaster or death of a loved one)

Sources: Stephen J. Servoss, James L. Januzzi, and James E. Muller, "Triggers of acute coronary syndromes," *Progress in Cardiovascular Diseases* 44, no. 5 (2002): 369–380; and Imre Janszky and Rickard Ljung, "Shifts to and from daylight saving time and incidence of myocardial infarction," *New England Journal of Medicine* 359, no. 18 (2008): 1966–1968.

into the blood calling all clotting factors, and dead macrophages within the core of the plaque release their own brand of a potent blood-clotting chemical called *tissue factor.*[16] Within one or two minutes, this massive exchange of blood and plaque components and clotting factors triggers the formation of a huge blood clot, a *thrombus* (Figure 2.7). Blood clots are inextricably linked to the

Death of Heart Muscle

Shoulder area (edge) of thin, frail cap ruptures

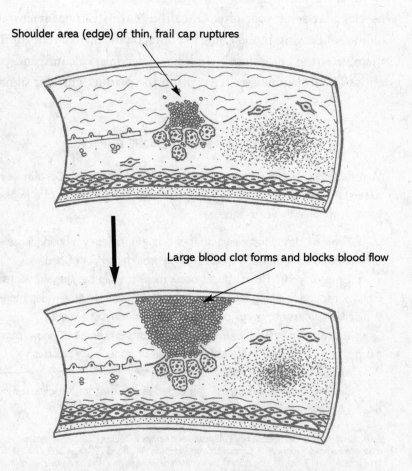

Large blood clot forms and blocks blood flow

Figure 2.7. The lethal step in most heart attack scenarios is the rupture of an unstable vulnerable plaque in a coronary artery and the formation of a large, occlusive blood clot. Cells downstream of the clot die.

heart attack scenario. One study found that 90 percent of people who experienced a fatal heart attack had evidence of thrombus formation.[17] (If you still haven't kicked the habit, you should know that cigarette smoking significantly increases the likelihood of a fatal blood clot, regardless of the type of vulnerable plaque. The chemicals in the smoke make the platelets in the blood stickier—hence clots form more easily, providing a compelling reason to break the smoking habit if you want to prevent another heart attack.)

Death of a heart muscle. Keep in mind that *it is not the plaque bursting that causes death*. Death of heart cells occurs because the blood does what it is supposed to do when it senses danger or broken vessels: It clots to stop the bleeding. The rupture of the plaque is recognized by the body as an injury; hence the blood clot is formed in an attempt to heal what is perceived as a wound (the fracture). If the clot (thrombus) enlarges enough to block the whole pipe, the flow of blood to the heart muscle (or in the case of a stroke, an artery to the brain) is cut off. When this happens, cells downstream do not receive oxygen or nutrients and they die; if the damage is great enough and enough cells die in your heart muscle, the result is a fatal heart attack.

KNOWLEDGE CAN HELP FIGHT ATHEROSCLEROSIS

In this chapter, you have learned about the intricate biology of atherosclerosis. This will help you understand how the preventive lifestyle strategies outlined in the Prevent a Second Heart Attack plan target the steps of the atherosclerotic process, thereby halting progression and even promoting regression of arterial plaque. In future chapters, you will see how in addition to your medication, the combination of certain foods and exercise in this book will help treat what scientists call the trilogy of vulnerability—the three greatest risk factors that impede your heart health. The Prevent a

Second Heart Attack plan will work in tandem with your medications to stabilize the following:

- Your vulnerable plaque—the high-risk, rupture-prone plaque (the type responsible for most heart attacks); following the plan will also reduce the likelihood that the plaque will burst, which could result in another and potentially fatal heart attack
- Your vulnerable blood—the composition of which is prone to form blood clots easily
- Your vulnerable heart muscle, which is prone to having an arrhythmia or electrical instability

But first, in the next chapter we'll look at the scientifically proven heart health benefits of the Prevent a Second Heart Attack plan's Mediterranean style of eating. Hundreds if not thousands of scientific studies reinforce the benefits of a diet high in olive oil, vegetables, fruits, fish, and nuts, and low in red meat and saturated fat. And once you start making the recipes in the back of this book, you'll find that the Mediterranean diet is as delicious as it is heart-healthy. This lifestyle will significantly reduce your risk of a second heart attack and help you live a longer, healthier, and happier life. Who in his or her right mind would trade this for a tasteless, low-fat deprivation diet?

The Science Behind the Solution

There are in fact two things, science and opinion;

the former begets knowledge, the latter ignorance.

—Hippocrates, Greek physician (460–377 B.C.)

The best long-term approach for preventing a second coronary event, medically called *secondary prevention,* is lifestyle change—diet and exercise—combined with smoking cessation, stress management, weight control, and the intensive drug therapy described in Chapter 2. Considering that you are at high risk for another heart attack by virtue of the fact that you have already survived one, I encourage you to consider applying all available strategies—paying particular attention to diet, exercise, medication, and stress management—to boost your protection against dying of a recurrent event. Because the main focus of this book is presenting the optimal lifestyle program to be used as an adjunct to your medication, let's first examine the scientific evidence that shows why this is the best, most practical diet for both the prevention and reversal of heart disease.

MEDITERRANEAN DIET: THE IDEAL HEALTHY-HEART DIET

The Mediterranean diet has been around for millennia, but only in recent decades have scientists begun to recognize it as the gold standard of healthy diets. For one thing, it is delectable—but perhaps more important, research proves that it has a favorable impact on health, quality of life, and longevity. It is described in the scientific literature as "very close to if not the ideal diet."[1]

Seven Countries Study proves diet and heart attack link

In 1958, Ancel Keys, a professor of physiology at the University of Minnesota School of Public Health, launched the famed Seven Countries Study.[2] Keys and a team of international scientists looked at the diets and rates of heart disease of 12,763 middle-aged men drawn from seven countries: Japan, Greece, Italy, the Netherlands, Yugoslavia, the United States, and Finland. The findings shocked the world. For the first time, it was shown that what human beings eat has a profound effect on their blood cholesterol level and subsequent risk of heart disease. No longer could heart disease be considered an inevitable consequence of aging. Countries such as Finland and the United States, where the men ate diets abundant in red meat and cheese—high in saturated fat—had much higher cholesterol and consequently sky-high rates of heart disease. This was in stark contrast to Greece and Japan, where the men consumed diets low in saturated fat and had low blood cholesterol levels and a significantly reduced rate of heart disease.

Keys's revolutionary line of thinking—that people's blood cholesterol level and risk of heart attack were greatly influenced by what was served at mealtimes—landed him on the cover of *Time* magazine in January 1961. Keys noticed that in the late 1950s and early 1960s, Greece had the highest life expectancy in the world and the lowest rate of coronary artery disease, suggesting that the eating habits of this population might be a model diet for promoting excellent health and longevity.

Interest in the eating habits of one group of Greek people in particular caught Keys's attention: the long-lived islanders of Crete. Keys and his wife, Margaret, went on to write a book, *How to Eat Well and Stay Well the Mediterranean Way,* in which Keys first used the term *good Mediterranean diet* to describe the traditional and extraordinarily healthful eating pattern of the Cretan people.[3] And so was born the concept of the Mediterranean diet.

EARLY STUDIES EXPLORE DIETS TO TREAT HEART DISEASE

Scientists took the findings from the Seven Countries Study and extrapolated that the best treatment for individuals with existing heart disease would be to place survivors on a low-saturated-fat diet. (Back then, researchers failed to look at the whole picture and did not differentiate between "good fats" and "bad fats.") Their goal was to generate data proving that a diet low in saturated fat and cholesterol would reduce blood cholesterol levels, thus preventing coronary relapses in individuals who had already experienced a heart attack.

The first generation of diet studies, called the *early studies,* consisted of three large trials conducted in the 1960s and 1970s in London, Sydney, and Oslo.[4] Following is an overview of these three early diet studies.

The Medical Research Council (MRC) Study

The MRC Study recruited 264 men from several London hospitals who had recently recovered from their first heart attack. The subjects were placed on either a control diet (their usual diet) or the experimental diet (called a "low-fat diet" by the researchers) for three years. Unsurprisingly, what was called "low fat" in 1965 London—in which the English breakfast (scrambled eggs, bacon, sausages, blood pudding, fried bread, mushrooms, and baked beans) and clotted cream were considered staples—is far from what dietitians would consider low-fat today. The experimental diet consisted of 45 grams of fat per day, with the average calorie intake of the experimental subjects at approximately 2000 calories per day—which means the diet was about 49 percent fat (albeit somewhat reduced in saturated fat because of substitution of full-fat milk with skim and other kinds of dietary saturated fat restrictions) compared to the control diet—which was also approximately 49 percent fat! The experimental group showed a decline in their blood cholesterol level of 10 percent, though the diet was poorly tolerated, as the subjects had a tough time sticking to it. The main objections were to the skim milk, the low butter ration, and the restriction on biscuits and cakes. Ultimately, the results were disappointing, because both the experimental group and the control group experienced the same rate of recurrent heart attacks and death.[5]

The Australian Low-Saturated-Fat, Low-Cholesterol Study

An Australian study put 458 men with heart disease on either a control diet or an experimental diet low in fat—although again, at 38 percent of total calories from fat, it was not what would be considered a "low-fat" diet today. (The diet was similar to the London study in that saturated fat was reduced by replacing butter—a highly saturated fat—with polyunsaturated margarine.) As in the MRC Study, the results were negative. Shockingly, after five years, the experimental group (the "low-fat" dieters) showed a slightly *lower* survival rate compared to the control group.[6]

The Oslo Heart Study

In Oslo, Norway, 412 male heart attack survivors were put on either a usual diet or the experimental "cholesterol-lowering diet." This eating pattern emulated the other first-generation diet studies in that the saturated fat was replaced with an extremely high amount of polyunsaturated fat in the form of linoleic acid—an omega-6 essential fat—found in high concentration in vegetable oils such as corn and safflower oil. After eleven years, researchers documented a 23 percent reduction in coronary events in the experimental group—yet there was no improvement in survival rate between groups. Despite the small trial size and less than spectacular results, the scientists *did* conclude that treating heart attack survivors with diet can reduce the occurrence of future coronary events.[7]

Early studies unsuccessful in extending longevity

Ultimately, these three early trials were all considered failures, because they did not help their patients live longer. All of the early studies used a low-saturated-fat diet similar to the one recommended by the American Heart Association at the time (the prudent National Cholesterol Education Program [NCEP]).[8] The three diets were comparable in that intake of saturated fat and cholesterol was restricted while consumption of polyunsaturated fat was increased. Thus, the common dietary characteristic in all three experimental groups was extremely high consumption of a type of polyunsaturated fat called linoleic acid. You will learn in Chapter 5 that the polyunsaturated fat linoleic acid is a pro-inflammatory food and is therefore *not* the best type of fat to replace saturated fat with, nor the type to ingest in large amounts for maximum cardio protection. Plus the fact that the trials were small, with fewer than 500 subjects in each, didn't help either—as the results are rendered less valid statistically by virtue of the small sample sizes. And so it was back to the drawing board for the scientists to figure out a better dietary strategy.

RECENT TRIALS SUPPORT MEDITERRANEAN-STYLE DIET'S HEALING POWER

Beginning in the 1980s, scientists began to revert back to Ancel Keys's concept of "the good Mediterranean diet" as a basis for constructing a better diet for secondary treatment of heart disease. Four more recent dietary trials evolved that all used a Mediterranean-style diet as the intervention, and the results were nothing short of spectacular. What's more, compared to the early research, the scientific design of these studies was much more valid—that is to say, the studies were better controlled—than those of the older trials. For example, the number of subjects recruited was much larger, the use of prescription drug therapy was meticulously recorded, and, most important, the subjects were better randomized. (Randomized clinical trials are the only way to ensure that the diet and not something else is responsible for the protective effect against heart disease.)

The Diet and Reinfarction Trial (DART)

The DART study was the first truly successful dietary trial to treat survivors of coronary artery disease (CAD). Conducted in 1989, the study recruited 2,033 men who had survived a heart attack. Although it did not test the "Mediterranean diet" per se, it did show the value of survivors' eating more fish and less saturated fat. Researchers placed the subjects in one of three groups, each receiving advice on different aspects of their diet: (1) the fat advice group, (2) the fish advice group, and (3) the fiber advice group. In the first group, subjects were instructed to reduce their total fat intake as well as change the proportions of the fat they ate, specifically by increasing polyunsaturated fat (especially the pro-inflammatory, omega-6 polyunsaturated fat found in margarine and vegetable oils) and reducing saturated fat. Subjects in the second group were advised to eat a lot of fatty fish, which is rich in the heart-healthiest type of polyunsaturated essential fat, the omega-3 fats. In the third group, subjects were told to eat a lot of fiber (increase fiber intake to at least 18 grams per day). After two years, the difference in deaths from all causes—not just heart disease—among the three groups was dramatic. The fish-eating group showed a 29 percent reduction in two-year death rates compared to the two other groups, which led scientists to an important conclusion: Giving *simple* dietary advice to eat a modest amount of fatty fish (two or three portions per week) can *cut the risk of death by 29 percent* in men during the first two years following a heart attack. Because two or three meals per week consisted of fish, that meant that two to three fewer meals consisted of meat, meat products, cheese, and eggs—all high in saturated fat—which may also have contributed to the higher survival rate.[9]

The Lyon Diet Heart Study

The researchers in the Lyon study decided to revert to the Seven Countries Study findings and construct a Cretan Mediterranean-style diet for recent heart attack survivors to follow. After a first heart attack, 605 men and women were randomly divided into two groups: the experimental diet group and the control group. Although no specific dietary advice was given to the control group, the subjects' physicians instructed them to follow a "prudent" cardiac diet similar to the NCEP Step I type of low-fat diet recommended by the AHA in the 1990s. Members of the experimental group were instructed to follow a Mediterranean-type diet rich in fruits, vegetables, grains, legumes, olive oil, fish (with very little red meat), and red wine with meals. This version of the Cretan Mediterranean diet also included an exceptionally large amount of a type of polyunsaturated fat called alpha-linolenic acid (ALA), an omega-3 fat (which you will learn much more about in Chapter 10) that is the precursor to the more physiologically active omega-3 fish fats DHA and EPA. After five years, the study results were remarkable. A *73 percent reduction* in risk of death from heart disease or a second heart attack was observed in the experimental group.[10] Clearly, these astonishing scientific findings provide striking evidence of the power of the Mediterranean diet and its proven ability to fend off future heart attacks in survivors of CAD.

The GISSI Prevention Trial

The GISSI (Gruppo Italiano per lo Studio della Sopravvivenza nell'Infarto Miocardico) Prevention Trial was a large Italian study involving 11,246 subjects and, similar to the Lyon study, was designed to find whether consumption of a Mediterranean-type diet lessens risk of death from CAD after a previous heart attack. A simple pamphlet describing suggested foods to include in the diet (fruits, vegetables, whole grains, olive oil, fish, legumes, fat-free dairy, poultry, and lean meats) was given to study participants. A five-food intake assessment (amounts of raw vegetables, cooked vegetables, fish, fruit, and olive oil) was calculated into a dietary score. Over the six-and-a-half-year duration of the study, dietary assessments were taken four times. Results revealed that the greater the subjects' adherence to the diet, the greater their chances of survival: A one-unit increase in the combined dietary score reduced the risk of death by 15 percent. Compared with subjects in the lowest quarter, those with the highest Mediterranean dietary score exhibited a *51 percent reduced risk of death*. As a result, the authors concluded that uncomplicated dietary advice to increase consumption of a few foods characteristic of the Mediterranean diet can lead to a substantial reduction in risk of death in patients having a history of a previous heart attack.[11]

The Indo-Mediterranean Diet Study

The first Indo-Mediterranean Diet Study was a randomized trial in the secondary prevention of CAD involving 406 South Asian patients who had just experienced a myocardial infarction.[12] Patients were assigned to their respective diet within twenty-four to forty-eight hours of having their heart attack. Subjects, most of whom were vegetarians, were randomized to an experimental Mediterranean-style diet rich in fruits, vegetables, and nuts. Subjects following the Mediterranean diet experienced significantly fewer cardiac complications, such as angina or electrical abnormalities, as well as dramatic declines in LDL cholesterol and triglycerides *after only six weeks on the diet.* After one year, a *42 percent reduction in risk of death from a cardiac event* was shown in subjects following the Mediterranean diet.

In a larger-scale follow-up of the Indo-Mediterranean Diet Study, researchers recruited 1,000 South Asian patients who had a previous diagnosis of CAD or were considered to be at high risk. Again, subjects were randomized to an experimental Mediterranean-style diet unusually high in ALA or a control diet similar to an NCEP Step I diet.[13] This version of the Mediterranean diet included ample fruits, vegetables, walnuts, whole grains, legumes, rice, maize, and wheat. After two years, *a 52 percent reduction in cardiac events* was shown in subjects following the Mediterranean diet supplemented with a high-ALA fat source (mustard seed or an ALA-rich oil). This study shows that including a significant amount of one particular type of fat—plant omega-3 ALA—in the Mediterranean diet appears to be a reasonable strategy for constructing an ideal cardioprotective eating plan, even if subjects are vegetarians.

HOW DO LOW-FAT DIETS COMPARE?

Despite the overwhelming scientific support for a relatively high-fat (albeit high in ultra-heart-healthy olive oil) and very appetizing Mediterranean style of eating for heart health, many health professionals still advocate a bland low-fat diet, and still others encourage extremely spartan vegetarian plans for treating heart disease patients. Are these deprivation diets better for cutting your risk of another attack? Let's see what the research says.

A more recent study published in 2006 in the *Archives of Internal Medicine* called the PREDIMED Study compared a traditional AHA low-fat diet with a Mediterranean-style diet and found that the Mediterranean diet was *superior* to the low-fat diet in re-ducing risk for heart disease.[14] Nine thousand subjects at high risk for heart disease across Spain participated in the study. After three months, the Mediterranean group exhibited lower levels of blood pressure, blood sugar, cho-lesterol, and triglycerides; fewer markers of inflammation; and an increase in HDL, or "good" cho-lesterol, compared to the low-fat group. These results support the Prevent a Second Heart Attack plan's contention that the optimal nutrition prescription for prevent-ing, treating, and reversing heart disease is a diet high in fruits, veg-etables, olive oil, whole grains, nuts, and fish—a relatively high-fat diet packed with protective nutrients including antioxidants, dietary fiber, and monounsaturated and omega-3 "good fats."

Take heart from the scientific research: It is not necessary for you to follow punishing, austere diet plans to prevent and reverse heart disease! A Mediterranean diet is superior to a low-fat one for promoting heart health and, thank goodness, is easier to swallow. Wine, olive oil, garlic, and chocolate . . . no deprivation here! This particular brand of the good life is good for you.

Foods of the Mediterranean Diet

What are the key foods that make up this ideal diet, and what about these foods makes them so spectacularly healthy? Researchers have found that the positive health effects of the Mediterranean diet are due not to individual nutrients or foods, but rather to the synergistic way these foods interact. Mediterranean cooking is like a symphony of foods; each of the delicious ingredients is a part of the healthy whole, and only when these "instruments" act together do we see the fantastic, heart-healthy effects.

The following chapters address the key foods that form the basis of this style of eating, foods that when consumed collectively provide a dietary pattern that is highly cardioprotective:

1. olive oil

2. greens

3. figs

4. omega-3 fish

5. walnuts and flaxseeds

6. lentils

7. oatmeal

8. red wine with meals and a small amount of dark chocolate (as a special bonus to you for all your heart-healing work!)

In the following chapters, you will learn how to use the Prevent a Second Heart Attack plan to craft delicious, simple recipes and incorporate them into daily meal plans. All the while, you will learn how exactly these foods target the trilogy of vulnerability by (1) stabilizing vulnerable plaque and reducing inflammation, (2) stabilizing the electrical conductivity of the heart muscle, and (3) changing the composition of the blood. As a bonus, you will also see how each individual food contributes to heart health by promoting lower blood pressure, resisting LDL oxidation, reducing your risk of diabetes (a major CAD risk factor), and decreasing arterial inflammation—all while adding vibrant years to your life.

The scientific data is clear: A Mediterranean diet is the best way to live a longer and fuller life, free of heart disease. All of us should take a culinary trip back in time to the Mediterranean countries of Greece and Italy during the 1960s—when their rates of heart disease were the lowest in the world and their longevity the longest—and learn from their healthy, happy lifestyles! Read on and start today to eat well, live well, and reap the astounding health benefits of this "good Mediterranean diet."

Part II

Reversing Heart Disease with Eight Foods and Exercise

Section 1

FOODS THAT HARM
THE ARTERIES

4

Beware the Plaque-Building Foods: Red Meat, Cream, Butter, Eggs, and Cheese

---

Every human being is the author of his own health or disease.

—Gautama Siddhartha, Hindu prince and founder of Buddhism (563–483 B.C.)

 Eat less than 15 grams of saturated fat, zero trans fat, and less than 200 milligrams of cholesterol every day.

Before you begin to enjoy the world's most healing foods, you need to know which foods in your diet can raise your risk of a second heart attack. So let's begin the "diet" section of this book by looking at the foods that make up the "Western" style of eating—the artery-clogging foods that got you into trouble in the first place.

As you're getting started, you must understand one important thing: The eight recommended foods discussed in this book are *not* a panacea. If you follow all the rules of the Prevent a Second Heart Attack plan but continue to eat foods that contain any or all of the three main dietary evils—saturated fat, trans fat, and dietary cholesterol—then you are sabotaging your hard work. These dietary land mines raise your level of circulating low-density lipoprotein (LDL) cholesterol—the type of cholesterol that initiates and promotes atherosclerosis as well as fuels inflammation. (Refer back to Chapter 2 for the major roles that both LDL and inflammation play in advancing heart disease.) What's more, many of the foods that contain these "bad fats" also work through other means to raise your risk of a second heart attack, such as increasing your triglyceride level, decreasing your "good" high-density lipoprotein (HDL) cholesterol, and contributing to metabolic syndrome (a disorder that increases your chances of developing diabetes and future heart disease events). You could exercise daily and regularly eat healthy portions of the plan's eight "miracle foods," but even that won't protect you from heart disease if you're still eating "bad" fats and cholesterol. This is why you *must* cut way back on your intake of foods that contain the most potent artery-clogging substances. So read on and learn why and how to substitute these dangerous foods with heart-protective choices that are also tasty and satisfying.

BAD FATS AND THE SEVEN COUNTRIES STUDY

As you learned in the previous chapter, pioneer nutrition researcher Dr. Ancel Keys (who passed away in 2004, two months before his 101st birthday) showed in his landmark Seven Countries Study just how powerful the connection between diet, cholesterol, and heart disease truly is.[1] Data from the early years of the study (1958–1964) revealed that in countries where people consumed foods high in saturated fat, there was a corresponding high level of blood cholesterol and a significantly higher rate of heart attack and stroke. Data obtained from the twenty-five-year follow-up went a step further, revealing that consumption of saturated fat significantly increases risk of *dying* of heart disease.[2] Intake of four major saturated fatty acids in particular—myristic, lauric, palmitic, and stearic acid—collectively had the strongest impact on death rates from heart disease. What's more, two additional types of fat, trans fat and dietary cholesterol, also significantly increased risk of death from the disease. Men from eastern Finland, the country with the highest twenty-five-year death rate from heart disease, ate an average of 89 grams of saturated fat, 5 grams of trans fat, and 537 milligrams of cholesterol per·day.

What's the take-away message? Saturated fat, trans fat, and dietary cholesterol each raise your blood cholesterol level and increase your risk of dying from a second heart attack.

HOW TO GIVE AN ANIMAL A HEART ATTACK

Scientists studying atherosclerosis in the laboratory usually induce the disease in healthy animals by adding a large amount of saturated fat and cholesterol to their lab animals' chow (in scientific terms, supplying the animals with an *atherogenic* diet). Certain types of monkeys, such as the rhesus monkey and the African green monkey, are frequently used in atherosclerosis research because of their humanlike physiology. When placed on diets high in saturated fat and cholesterol, these primates develop plaque in their coronary arteries in a remarkably similar fashion to the way humans develop plaque.

AIDS researchers at Harvard Medical School decided to test

BANISH THESE BAD FATS FROM YOUR DIET

Butter

Oils other than extra virgin olive oil, flaxseed oil, canola oil, and walnut oil

Any food containing coconut oil, palm oil, or palm kernel oil

Cream

Full-fat cheese in large amounts (occasional use of a small amount of strong cheese like Parmesan or Romano is okay)

Full-fat dairy products such as ice cream and whole milk

Egg yolks

Red meat and processed meats

Commercial baked goods (in restaurants, or boxed and bagged convenience foods)

Commercial fried foods

Packaged or processed foods with trans fat or the word *hydrogenated* or *shortening* in the ingredients list the effects of diet on disease progression in primates by comparing two groups of rhesus monkeys—one group was fed an atherogenic diet (that is to say, high in saturated fat and cholesterol), and the other was fed a normal diet.[3] Not surprisingly, monkeys on the atherogenic diet developed atherosclerosis in their arteries, as well as increased blood cholesterol levels, triglycerides, and markers of inflammation. But they also had an accelerated HIV disease course, and scientists concluded that a diet high in cholesterol and saturated fat promotes atherosclerosis and inflammation, which accelerates the progression of HIV. The take-away message (as it applies to you) from this study is to confirm what hundreds of animal studies have concluded already—the greater your intake of dietary saturated fat, the higher your level of "bad" LDL cholesterol and the greater your odds of "clogging up."

A QUICK LESSON IN FAT CHEMISTRY

On a molecular level, the main ingredient of any fat—be it butter, cream, or olive oil—is triglyceride molecules (Figure 4.1). Each triglyceride molecule is made up of a glycerol backbone that supports three fatty acid chains. The chemical makeup of each of these fatty acid chains dictates how the fat will behave once it is digested and enters your body. There are three types of chains, or fatty acids. Scientists have named the three types *saturated, monounsaturated,* and *polyunsaturated.* The different types of chains can exist in different combinations in each triglyceride molecule, and the *predominant* type of chain helps scientists categorize fats as either saturated, monounsaturated, or polyunsaturated. For example, about half the fatty acid chains in palm oil (an inexpensive tropical oil used in many processed foods) are saturated, plus 45 percent of those saturated fatty acids are composed of palmitic acid—an extremely artery-damaging type of saturated fatty acid.

Not all fats (or fatty acids) are created equal. Saturated fat is

Triglycerides Make Up the Fat We Eat

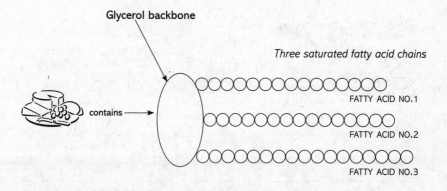

Figure 4.1. Triglycerides are three-chain molecules that make up most of the fat we eat. Saturated fat refers to one type of "chain," or fatty acid, that dangles off the triglyceride's backbone. Beef, cheese, and butter contain triglycerides with a large percentage of saturated fatty acid chains linked to the glycerol backbone.

one of the most dangerous foods you can eat in terms of promoting heart disease, so understanding the difference between the healthy and the unhealthy fats is important.

Unhealthy fats

Unhealthy fats fall into two basic categories: saturated fat and synthetic trans fat.

Saturated fat. If the fat has a large percentage of shorter, straight chains in the triglyceride molecules, then the fat is called *saturated* and often appears solid at room temperature (due to the straight shape of the fatty acid chains, which allows them to be closely packed together). Large amounts of saturated fatty acids are found in butter, meats, full-fat dairy foods, and tropical oils (Figure 4.2). Saturated fat raises your blood level of bad LDL cholesterol. Furthermore, saturated fat becomes incorporated within the LDL

Saturated "Bad" Fat

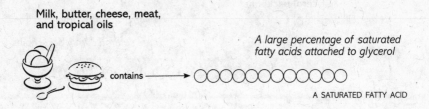

Milk, butter, cheese, meat,
and tropical oils

*A large percentage of saturated
fatty acids attached to glycerol*

contains ⟶ A SATURATED FATTY ACID

Figure 4.2. Butter is not better. Saturated fat is found in foods of animal origin such as meat, butter, whole milk, cream, and cheese. Saturated fat is also found in vegetable oils such as coconut, palm kernel, and palm oil.

cholesterol particles circulating in your blood, increasing your LDL's ability to participate in plaque formation in the coronary arteries.

Interestingly, no naturally occurring fat or oil contains fatty acid chains that are completely saturated. In fact, all fats or oils are made up of a combination of all three types of fatty acids: saturated, monounsaturated, and polyunsaturated. The trick is to choose the fats and oils that contain the lowest percentage of artery-clogging saturated fat and the greatest percentage of artery-healing mono-unsaturated or polyunsaturated fatty acids (omega-3). For example, most of the triglyceride molecules in the beef fat dripping off your burger contain the shorter-chain, "bad" cholesterol–raising fatty acids, typically large numbers of palmitic acid, the exceptionally artery-clogging sixteen-carbon saturated fatty acid discussed previously. Hence, beef is a chief source of saturated fat—roughly 51 percent of beef fat is made up of saturated fatty acids. Some other fats and oils that have the highest percentages of saturated fatty acids are coconut oil (77 percent), butter fat (54 percent), and lard (pork fat; 42 percent). The nutritionist's rule of thumb is that if the fat is hard at room temperature, it is considered a bad, or saturated, fat.

Trans fat. Trans fat is created when food manufacturers turn a liquid polyunsaturated vegetable oil into a solid fat by a chemical process called *hydrogenation*. This procedure rearranges the shape of the fatty acid chains, straightening out the slightly bent chains so they can fit side by side, closer together, similar to straight saturated fatty acids, and making the fat more stable and more solid (Figure 4.3). Trans fats, even if consumed in small portions, fuel the progression of atherosclerosis. The bottom line is, it is never safe to eat trans fats, so stay away at all cost!

Trans "Bad" Fat

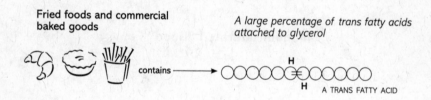

Fried foods and commercial baked goods

A large percentage of trans fatty acids attached to glycerol

contains →

A TRANS FATTY ACID

Figure 4.3. Trans fat hardens fats as well as arteries. Potent food sources of trans fat include fast and frozen foods (French fries, pot pies); commercially baked or processed foods (doughnuts, cakes, pies); packaged snacks (microwave popcorn, chips); margarines and shortening; pancakes; and crackers.

Healthy fats (unsaturated fats)

Unsaturated fatty acids are mostly "good," or protective, fats, found in plants such as nuts, seeds, and olives or in marine life (fatty.

fish). Healthy, unsaturated fats fall into two categories: monounsaturated and polyunsaturated.

Monounsaturated. Unsaturated fatty acids have longer chains than saturated fatty acids and also contain varying numbers of double bonds, or "kinks," in the long fatty acid chain. If the chain contains only one kink, or one spot of unsaturation, it is called a *monounsaturated* fatty acid. Fats that contain a large percentage of monounsaturated fatty acids include olive oil, avocados, and most nuts (Figure 4.4).

Polyunsaturated. There are two classes of polyunsaturated fatty acids: omega-3 and omega-6. Both types of fatty acids contain several kinks, or spots of unsaturation, in the chain—multiple double bonds where a carbon is missing two hydrogen atoms. Thus, they are referred to as *polyunsaturated*. The multiple double bonds

Monounsaturated "Good" Fat

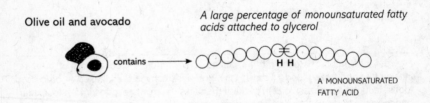

Olive oil and avocado

A large percentage of monounsaturated fatty acids attached to glycerol

contains ⟶

H H

A MONOUNSATURATED
FATTY ACID

Figure 4.4. Monounsaturated fat heals the arteries. The Prevent a Second Heart Attack plan recommends liberal use of extra virgin olive oil, the earth's richest source of heart-healthy monounsaturated fat, and other foods high in monounsaturated fats such as avocado.

allow these unsaturated fats to have bends in their structure—enabling the fatty acids to favor hook shapes—which limits their ability to be closely packed together and solid at room temperature like saturated fat. Liquid unsaturated fatty acids tend to be heart-healthier than solid saturated fats. As you will soon learn, one particular type of polyunsaturated fatty acid, the omega-3s, are the most cardioprotective. A large concentration of omega-3 fatty acids is found in fatty fish such as salmon and in plant foods such as flaxseeds (Figure 4.5).

If the fat is liquid at room temperature, a large percentage of the fatty acid chains on the triglyceride molecules are long and the fat tends to be "good." For example, olive oil has the largest percentage (about 77 percent) of the monounsaturated fatty acid oleic acid, whereas flaxseed oil has the largest percentage (roughly 53 percent) of the polyunsaturated omega-3 fatty acid alpha-linolenic acid.

Polyunsaturated "Good" Fat

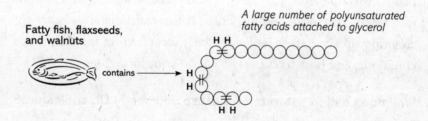

Fatty fish, flaxseeds, and walnuts

contains →

A large number of polyunsaturated fatty acids attached to glycerol

AN OMEGA-3 POLYUNSATURATED FATTY ACID

Figure 4.5. Polyunsaturated fat can be healthful and harmful. The Prevent a Second Heart Attack plan recommends liberal use of anti-inflammatory polyunsaturated fats, the essential omega-3 fatty acids found in fish, flaxseeds, and nuts.

WHICH FATS BELONG IN YOUR KITCHEN?

Good: extra virgin olive oil, canola oil, flaxseed oil, almond oil

OK: walnut oil, sesame oil, peanut oil

Not so good: corn oil, safflower oil, cottonseed oil, sunflower oil

Bad: butter, lard, hydrogenated (trans) fats, tropical oils (palm oil, palm kernel oil, coconut oil)

The best advice in the kitchen is to replace plaque-building or inflammatory fats—butter, hydrogenated fats, and tropical oils—with healthful oils containing a low amount of saturated fatty acids and a relatively high amount of the heart-healthy fatty acids: monounsaturated fatty acids and omega-3 fatty acids.

SATURATED FAT: THE MAIN DIETARY CAUSE OF HIGH CHOLESTEROL

Saturated fat is probably the worst offender of the three bad fats in terms of raising LDL levels and promoting inflammation because Americans *eat so much of it*. We eat it in steaks, in butter, in ice cream, in milk, in cream cheese, in bacon, and in our eggs, to name just a few. Saturated fat is doubly risky for heart attack survivors because it not only raises LDL cholesterol but also increases insulin secretion from the pancreas. Increased insulin secretion can often lead to insulin resistance, which in turn promotes the metabolic syndrome thought to precede the development of diabetes. (If you're wondering why this matters, consider this statistic: Two out of three people with diabetes will die of a heart attack or stroke.) The bottom line is that saturated fat intake is the main dietary trigger for clogging up your arteries. Know what saturated fat is, what foods contain it, and how to cut way back on your intake.

Why does eating saturated fat cause your bad LDL cholesterol to go up?

According to nutrition scientists at Pennsylvania State University,[4] saturated fatty acids raise LDL because they slow the activity of cholesterol receptors on liver cells. LDL liver receptors are the clearinghouse for blood LDL cholesterol. In a nutshell, the receptors catch all the excess LDL cholesterol that is swimming through the bloodstream, then transfer it to the liver, where it is processed and then excreted. Less LDL receptor activity means less LDL cleared from the bloodstream and a higher blood level, which as we now know fuels atherosclerosis. In addition to increasing your levels of bad cholesterol, saturated fat can also hinder the ability of good HDL cholesterol to control blood vessel inflammation. Recall from Chapter 2 that an inflamed endothelium (the inner layer of the coronary artery) is a key early event in the process of atherosclerosis. A study published in the *Journal of the American College of Cardiology* revealed that just one meal high in saturated fat reduces the anti-inflammatory potential of HDL and promotes endothelial dysfunction.[5] Therefore, an overdose of saturated fat—even if you eat it just once during the day—raises the amount of LDL in the bloodstream, reduces the anti-inflammatory effect of HDL, and triggers plaque formation. The message should be clear: Pass on that buttery biscuit or fatty steak!

> ### THE BAD SIDE OF BUTTER
>
> Butter is loaded with saturated fatty acids. Scientists have determined that saturated fats propel atherosclerosis in a variety of ways:
>
> - Elevate "bad" LDL cholesterol
> - Increase the blood's ability to form clots
> - Impair the function of the endothelial layer of the coronary arteries, fueling inflammation
> - Increase oxidative stress
>
> Switch to heart-healthy extra virgin olive oil in place of butter and you will be taking a major step toward slowing plaque buildup in your arteries.
>
> *Source:* Robert Vogel et al., "The postprandial effect of components of the Mediterranean diet on endothelial function," *Journal of the American College of Cardiology* 36, no. 5 (2000): 1455–1460.

We know that eating a diet high in saturated fat promotes heart disease. But what if you've already been diagnosed with heart disease? What can switching to a Mediterranean diet—extremely low in saturated fat—do to reverse the heart disease process and stop that second and potentially fatal heart attack? Researchers out of the Netherlands experimented with just this question. When heart disease patients were put on a Cretan-style Mediterranean diet exceptionally low in saturated fat, the researchers reported *a 70 percent lower death rate* in those following the Mediterranean diet compared to those adhering to the control diet.[6]

LOWERING LDL LOWERS RISK OF A SECOND HEART ATTACK

High LDL cholesterol initiates and promotes atherosclerosis. Eating foods with saturated fat, trans fat, or cholesterol can increase your LDL cholesterol level. Reduce your intake of these foods and your LDL will drop, thereby cutting your risk of having another heart attack. In fact, for every 1.8 mg/dL reduction in LDL cholesterol, you lower your risk of having another "cardiac event" (heart attack, stroke, or hospitalization for unstable angina—a condition that precludes a heart attack) by approximately 1 percent. That means if you get your LDL down from, say, 100 mg/dL to 70 mg/dL, you cut your risk by almost 20 percent. The best way to get that LDL down is to take a three-pronged approach:

1. Take your statin medication.
2. Follow the ten lifestyle steps outlined in my previous book, *Cholesterol Down*.
3. Switch to the Mediterranean-inspired Prevent a Second Heart Attack eating plan very low in saturated fat, trans fat, and cholesterol.

Source: C. P. Cannon et al., "Meta-analysis of cardiovascular outcomes trials comparing intensive versus moderate statin therapy," *Journal of the American College of Cardiology* 48, no. 3 (2006): 438–445.

What food contains saturated fat?

Not to be confused with dietary cholesterol, which comes only from animals, saturated fat is found in *both* animal and plant products. The following foods contain large amounts of artery-clogging saturated fat:

- Fatty cuts of beef and pork (think ribs, sausage, and bacon)
- Full-fat dairy products (such as premium ice cream or a slab of Cheddar cheese)

- butter (such as what you may slather on your baked potatoes, toast, and corn)
- tropical oils (coconut oil or palm kernel oil hidden in foods such as oil-roasted nuts and processed, packaged foods)
- lard (found in refried beans and baked foods)
- fast food (think cheeseburger and fries or that diner breakfast special of scrambled eggs, sausage, biscuit, and hotcakes)

Animal foods provide most of the saturated fat in our diet. The top source of saturated fat in the American diet is red meat—especially the ground beef in that all-American favorite, hamburger—and full-fat dairy products.[7] If you haven't figured it out already . . . these are foods to stay away from!

Can I eat *any* saturated fat?

The Institute of Medicine suggests that Americans keep intake of saturated fat as low as possible. If you're interested in keeping track of numbers, the government's National Cholesterol Education Program (NCEP) recommends that for a therapeutic diet designed specifically to lower LDL cholesterol, one should consume less than 7 percent of total daily calories from saturated fat[8]; that is to say, less than 15 grams of saturated fat per 2,000 calories. (FYI, a McDonald's Double Quarter Pounder with cheese contains 19 grams of saturated fat.) In addition to high-fat proteins such as hot dogs or ground beef, cheese is a top source of saturated fat in the American diet. I know that cutting out cheese might seem like a tall order—especially considering how much we Americans love our pizza! But here's a heart-healthy tip: Try ordering pizza and other prepared foods without the cheese—add in veggies instead. For extra flavor, lightly sprinkle on Parmesan cheese and you'll be treating yourself to a more healthful but still tasty meal.

The simplest approach for lowering saturated fat intake is to scan Nutrition Facts panels and don't eat foods with more than

FOODS HIGH IN SATURATED FAT

Food	Saturated Fat (grams)*
Cheddar cheese, 3 ounces	18
Bacon cheeseburger	16
Coconut, 1 piece (2" × 2" × ½)	13
Lard/shortening, 2 tablespoons	10
Ice cream, 1 cup	10
Fried chicken with skin, 3.5 ounces	8
Butter, 1 tablespoon	7
Whole milk, 12 fluid ounces	7

*Saturated fat goal: less than 15 grams per day.

1 or 2 grams of saturated fat per serving. Because animal foods provide most of the saturated fat in the American diet, and saturated fat is the most potent LDL-raising substance, your best strategy is to *eat more plants and fewer animal-based foods.*

TRANS FAT: MORE HARMFUL THAN SATURATED FAT?

Trans fatty acids, commonly referred to as trans fat, are a synthetic mutant fat that could soon replace saturated fat as the most dangerous fat in American foods. Although it isn't as common in our diets as saturated fat, it is far more deadly, which is why you should be on a special lookout for trans fats on nutrition labels.

How is trans fat created?

The cheapest and most abundant source of fat is plant oil, and natural, unsaturated oils are liquid in nature. But liquid, unsaturated plant oils do not keep well, nor do they add much flavor to processed foods—which is why food companies worked to develop an artificial, solid type of fat that would boost shelf life and taste good in baked commercial goods. Scientists came up with a great solution. Change the chemical structure of cheap liquid vegetable oil by adding hydrogen—a process called *hydrogenation*—and voilà, what was once a healthful liquid oil is now a partially solidified fat, perfect for baking. What's more, the new partially hydrogenated fat makes the cookies taste great and allows them to sit on the shelf for long time periods without going rancid. The extra hydrogen pumped in makes the fat somewhat softer, too, so the cookies stay nice and moist. Cookie companies aren't the only ones using these oils, though—those deep-fried nachos or French fries you just ordered at the drive-through were also cooked in industrially produced trans fat. Because this oil doesn't go rancid as easily, it can withstand deep-frying for extended periods and can be reused for a longer time than conventional oils—saving the restaurateur a pretty penny on frying fats. Good for the food manufacturers and restaurant owners, bad for the consumer.

Because of public backlash against trans fat, several restaurants and fast-food establishments have switched to frying oils with 0 grams of trans fat. The American Heart Association, working with the Trans Fat Help Center in New York City, provides suggestions for switching to trans-fat-free fats and oils and supplies a list of products with 0 grams of trans fat at http://www.americanheart .org/presenter.jhtml?identifier=3050715.

How bad is trans fat?

It turns out that just like saturated fat and dietary cholesterol, trans fat raises your LDL. Keep in mind that trans fat is chemically different from saturated fat. Saturated fat is by far the more potent LDL-raising dietary fat, but that's just because we eat four to five times as much of it as we do trans fat. But trans fat may be worse for you because it not only raises LDL but also lowers your good HDL cholesterol—the substance that keeps the amount of LDL in check—so you have twice the negative effect.

Not only does trans fat increase the quantity of LDL in the blood, but it can also change the shape of the LDL particles. New research reveals that trans fat can morph the makeup of the LDL particle from fat and fluffy to small and dense (the dangerous kind). Researchers at Tufts University showed that the more trans fat subjects ate, the greater the reduction in LDL particle size.[9] Additional research has found that trans fat increases inflammation in the arteries, increases the risk of type 2 diabetes, and raises triglycerides as well as another type of dangerous blood fat, Lp(a), each of which further elevates the risk of heart disease.[10]

THE TROUBLE WITH TRANS

Researchers have discovered that individuals with the highest level of trans fatty acids in their cell membranes have a four times greater risk of having a heart attack and two and one-half times the risk of having a fatal cardiac event compared to individuals with the lowest level of trans fatty acids. Another major review on the health effects of trans fat concluded that on a per-calorie basis, trans fat increases risk of heart disease more than any other nutrient. A 2 percent increase in calorie intake from trans fat was associated with a 23 percent increase in new cases of heart disease. Concern over dietary trans fatty acids has led some scientists to state that trans fat is more deleterious in promoting heart disease than even saturated fatty acids.

Sources: Heather I. Katcher et al., "Lifestyle approaches and dietary strategies to lower LDL-cholesterol and triglycerides and raise HDL-cholesterol," *Endocrinology Metabolism Clinics North America* 38 (2009): 45–78; Dariush Mozaffarian et al., "Trans fatty acids and cardiovascular disease," *New England Journal of Medicine* (2006) 345: 1601–1603; and Alberto Ascherio et al., "Trans fatty acids and coronary heart disease," *New England Journal of Medicine* 340, no. 25 (1999): 1994–1998.

What foods contain trans fat?

According to the U.S. Food and Drug Administration (FDA) ruling on trans fatty acid labeling (July 11, 2003),[11] the main source of trans fat in the American diet is commercial baked goods such as cakes, pies, doughnuts, sweet rolls, biscuits, muffins, pancakes, and quick breads, followed by cookies and crackers. French fries, chips, and popcorn also are generally loaded with deadly trans fat. Animal products such as fast-food fried chicken and potpies contain appreciable amounts of trans fat, as do margarines, particularly stick margarine.

Effective January 1, 2006, the government required that all

food manufacturers list trans fat on the Nutrition Facts panel directly underneath the saturated fat line. So be vigilant about reading those labels! Note that if the food label boasts "trans fat free," it may still contain trans fat. The law states that if the product contains less than 0.5 grams of trans fat per serving, the label can still make the trans-fat-free claim. However, many people eat far more than one serving. Get around this loophole by scanning the ingredients list. If you see the words *hydrogenated, partially hydrogenated,* or *shortening,* return the product to the shelf.

Seems other countries are ahead of the United States in terms of policing trans fat in processed food. In 2003, Denmark instituted a ban on all products containing more than 2 percent trans fat for every 100 grams of fat. Switzerland followed suit, implementing a ban on trans fat in April 2008. Here in the United States, a select few cities have banned the use of this type of modified fat in restaurants. At the time of this writing, thirteen cities in the United States and Puerto Rico, such as New York City, Philadelphia, and Boston, have banned trans fats in restaurants.

Slowly but surely, we are starting to get the trans fat out of our food supply. Major U.S. food manufacturers have cut trans fat from hundreds of lines of foods, a complex and expensive process to modify products without affecting taste. As a result, today consumers do have more choices of trans-fat-free foods. According to the Center for Science in the Public Interest, "The amount of trans fat being put in our food has declined by 50 percent since about 2005."[12]

So what's the best way to ensure that you are cutting trans fat

FOODS HIGH IN TRANS FAT

Food	Trans Fat (grams)*
Fast-food fries (king-size serving)	10.0
Stick margarine, 2 tablespoons	6.0
Commercial doughnut	5.0
Pancake or cake mix, 1 cup	4.5
Commercial apple pie, 1 slice	4.0
Commercially baked cookies, 2	2.5

*Trans fat goal: zero intake per day.

out of your life? Stay away from fast and processed foods, read labels, and do your frying and baking at home using healthful fat, such as olive oil and canola oil, or try replacing some of the fat in baking with fruit purée.

How much trans fat should you eat?

None, if possible. Clear and to the point, when trans fat intake goes down, deaths from coronary artery disease go down. The National Academy of Sciences has concluded that *there is no safe level of trans fat consumption.*[13] There is a reason why there is no recommended daily allowance of trans fat on nutrition panels: Trans fat is a threat to public health.

DIETARY CHOLESTEROL: LESS IS BETTER FOR YOUR ARTERIES

The third of the three dietary evils is cholesterol. Cholesterol is not a fatty acid like saturated fat or trans fat but a different type of fat—one that, when created naturally in our own bodies, is vital for life. The body uses cholesterol for multiple functions such as building cell walls, producing steroid hormones, and making bile acids for digestion, and as a starting point for vitamin D formation. Our livers make all the cholesterol we need, though (the average person manufactures about 800 milligrams of cholesterol a day), so any cholesterol that we *ingest* is potentially dangerous overkill.

Cholesterol is one more fat you definitely want to eat less of. Once again, an abundance of scientific evidence has demonstrated that *diets high in cholesterol raise LDL levels, increase plaque formation, and contribute to atherosclerosis.* A recent study out of the Netherlands linked dietary cholesterol to severe inflammation in the liver, which eventually led to plaque formation in the animal subjects' hearts. Additional animal research has revealed that when the cholesterol we eat goes through a chemical process called *oxidation* (it comes into contact with oxygen and decomposes—

A QUICK WORD ON SALT: THE SLOW POISON

Salt is a vital nutrient required for the body to function properly. However, we eat far too much salt in Westernized countries, which according to the Consensus Action on Salt and Health (CASH) averages about 10 to 12 grams per day. Too much salt contributes to the development of high blood pressure—a leading risk factor for heart disease. Even a mildly elevated blood pressure harms the arteries. Individuals with a blood pressure of 130/85 or greater have twice the risk of experiencing a heart attack than those with a blood pressure of less than 120/80. The World Health Organization recommends a daily intake of just 5 grams to prevent and control high blood pressure. (One gram of salt contains about 400 milligrams of sodium. The American Heart Association recommends that middle-aged and older adults and people with high blood pressure consume *less than 1500 milligrams of sodium* per day.) A recent study published in the *British Medical Journal* of a group of individuals with borderline to high blood pressure found that cutting back on their salt intake diminished their risk of contracting heart disease by 25 percent and of dying of the disease by up to 20 percent. The researchers surmised that sodium acts directly on the blood vessel walls, stiffening them and making them more susceptible to atherosclerosis. The American Public Health Association has called for a 50 percent reduction in the amount of sodium in food in the United States. To reduce your sodium intake, you should know that 75 percent of the daily intake of sodium comes from both processed and restaurant foods. So learn to read those labels, cook at home, and order food in restaurants wisely.

Sources: American Heart Association, "Recommendation on sodium intake," http://www.americanheart .org/presenter.jhtml?identifier=4708; and Nancy R. Cook et al., "Long-term effects of dietary sodium reduction on cardiovascular disease outcomes: Observational follow-up of the trials of hypertension prevention (TOHP)," *British Medical Journal* (2007): doi:10.1136/bmj.39147.604896.55.

similar to when metal rusts), the resulting oxidized cholesterol contributes to fatty streak formation and atherosclerosis.[14] Researchers originally discovered this by feeding oxidized cholesterol to rabbits, and when they fed the same oxidized cholesterol to humans with diabetes, they found that the damaging fats became a part of the subject's bloodstream. This is important to understand, particularly if you are diabetic, as high levels of oxidized cholesterol in your

blood for an extended period of time following a meal will accelerate plaque growth in your arteries. Recall that people with diabetes
are in grave danger of dying from heart disease. All Americans,
however, should beware: We consume a large amount of oxidized
cholesterol in our daily diets. Food processing, especially heat treatment of foods naturally high in cholesterol, such as some breakfast
favorites like fried bacon, sausage, and eggs, produces the more
artery-clogging, oxidized version of dietary cholesterol.

What foods contain cholesterol?

There's an old saying among nutritionists: "If it had a mother or a
face, it has cholesterol." Cholesterol is found only in the cells of animals; meat, chicken, fish, milk products, and eggs all contain cholesterol. The fat portion of milk products harbors the cholesterol,
so if you switch to fat-free dairy products, you eliminate a prime dietary source of cholesterol. Forget the pâté—large amounts of cholesterol are found in organ meats such as liver. Even as little as 3
ounces of chicken liver contains an astounding 537 milligrams.

How much cholesterol should you eat?

The NCEP recommends that individuals trying to lower LDL
through dietary means should consume no more than 200 milligrams of cholesterol per day.[15] Just as with saturated fat, when it
comes to cholesterol . . . less is better!

Cholesterol is different from fat. If you cut off the fatty edge of
a slab of beef, you still have cholesterol. That's because both the
lean portion and the fatty cuts of meat or poultry (dark and light,
skin on or off) contain similar amounts of cholesterol. Remember
that cholesterol is found in large quantities in the membranes or
casings of animal cells. Considering that all animal protein sources
contain cholesterol, and that reducing cholesterol intake is the
goal, why not include several nights of vegetarian dinners in your
menu plan? Plant foods are naturally cholesterol-free yet contain a

sizable array of essential amino acids, the building blocks of protein. Frequently substituting plant-based meals for animal-based meals not only will lower cholesterol, it will also provide a healthful source of essential protein.

Another tip for lowering cholesterol intake is to routinely eat fish over all other animal protein choices. The beauty of fish is that it's a great protein source, contains much less cholesterol and saturated fat than meat, and has heart-healthy omega-3 fatty acids not found in meat or chicken. Even though shellfish such as shrimp is fairly high in cholesterol (166 milligrams in 3 ounces), a small portion allows you to stay under your maximum daily limit (200 milligrams per day), plus it contains heart-healthy omega-3 fats and only a negligible amount of saturated fat, so it would still be a better choice than beef.

Should you eat eggs?

The great egg debate . . . should we limit eggs in our diet and do they really raise cholesterol? This has been a topic of contention in the nutrition world for years. Newer analyses have found that eggs contain less cholesterol than previously thought: 213 to 220 milligrams, not 275 milligrams. Moreover, eggs are low in saturated fat and full of healthy nutrients such as protein, iron, zinc, B vitamins, vitamin D, and vitamin E. Keep in mind, however, that eggs are a high-cholesterol food and that all the cholesterol is located in the yolk. Egg whites contain high-quality protein and are very low in calories (one large egg white contains 17 calories and 4 grams of protein), so if you choose to eat eggs, make sure to chuck the yolks first, then go ahead and eat your whites with abandon!

Scientists have questioned the impact that eating eggs has on raising the risk of heart disease. Some studies suggest that dietary cholesterol (consumed in the form of eggs) has a marked effect on risk for heart disease, whereas others find no significant association between egg consumption and increased risk. New research has shown a wide variation in an individual's response to eating eggs (dietary cholesterol), which may reflect a strong genetic component. Some individuals can eat all the cholesterol-rich foods they want and exhibit no change in their LDL cholesterol levels. Remember, one egg yolk contains between 213 and 220 milligrams of cholesterol, so eat just one and you've well exceeded the recommended maximum intake of 200 milligrams per day by the NCEP. Another problem with eggs is that they are hidden in many of the foods we consume, such as pancakes, breads, sauces, and desserts. Combine the cholesterol derived from those foods with the one or two egg yolks you may consciously consume and you are way over your cholesterol limit. For example, eat just one egg for breakfast, a 4-ounce turkey sandwich with mayonnaise for lunch, and a 6-ounce veal chop for dinner, and your daily dietary cholesterol tally is at about 500 milligrams. Considering that eggs contribute approximately one third of the cholesterol in our food supply,[16] I say, play it safe! If you choose to eat eggs, toss the yolks and zero in on the whites and egg substitutes, which are a heart-healthier option.

FOODS HIGH IN DIETARY CHOLESTEROL

Food	Cholesterol (milligrams)*
Organ meats, 3.5 ounces	400–600
Egg yolk	220
Shrimp, 3.5 ounces	195
Chicken meat, 3.5 ounces, cooked	80
Fish, white, 3.5 ounces, cooked	70
Butter, 1 tablespoon	30

*Cholesterol goal: less than 200 milligrams per day. Plant foods—fruits, vegetables, beans, grains, nuts, and seeds—contain zero cholesterol, so replace animal foods with plant foods when possible to reduce dietary cholesterol intake.

YOU ARE WHAT YOU DON'T EAT

Thanks to the groundbreaking research by Dr. Ancel Keys, we now know that not all fats are equal in terms of their effect on heart disease risk. Keys noted that where we come from has a great deal to do with the type of fats we eat: Northern Europeans ate butter, lard, and beef tallow, whereas southern Europeans ate primarily olive oil. Consequently, people in the north had five times the death rate from heart disease of people in the south.[17] Inhabitants of the Mediterranean basin in particular, whose diets were rich in fruits, vegetables, nuts, whole grains, fish, and olive oil (a monounsaturated fat), but low in meat, milk, and cheese (potent sources of saturated fat), exhibited the lowest rates of cardiovascular disease and the greatest longevity of any group in the world.

The key point to remember is that what you eat can greatly accelerate plaque buildup in your arteries—and what you don't eat can drastically lower your intake of bad fats and greatly reduce your odds of another cardiac event. To prevent and reverse heart disease, you will need to work on decreasing your consumption of the three dietary villains—saturated fat, trans fat, and dietary cholesterol—so that you can start to reap the benefits of the Prevent a Second Heart Attack plan.

But enough about what you *can't* eat—let's start talking about all the delicious foods you can and *should* add to your daily meals. We'll take a lesson from the long-lived Greek islanders, who were known for savoring the pleasures of eating while leading long and healthy lives. Read on to see how you, too, can cook minimally processed and seasonally fresh fare—using fantastic, affordable ingredients and flavorful, nutritious fats from plant oils, nuts, and seeds. If you're tired of depriving yourself of the foods you love most, how does this menu sound for a change: fresh fish grilled simply with a dash of olive oil, lemon, and herbs for protein; lentils, beans, nuts, and grains for fiber; local, seasonal vegetables and fruit for disease-fighting antioxidants; and all washed down with a pleasing, heart-healthy glass of red wine and some dark chocolate for dessert. Is your mouth watering yet? If so, read on!

Section 2

FOODS THAT HEAL
THE ARTERIES

5

Heart-Healthy Food Number 1: Extra Virgin Olive Oil

He that takes medicine and neglects diet wastes the skill of the physician.

—Chinese proverb

 Consume 2 tablespoons of extra virgin olive oil every day, making this your main, and preferably your sole added fat.

Companion foods Rx: avocado and natural, dry-roasted almonds
Primary disease-fighting bioactive compounds:

- Monounsaturated fatty acid—oleic acid
- Polyphenol compounds—hydroxytyrosol, tyrosol, oleuropein
- Vitamin E

The centerpiece of the Mediterranean style of eating is olive oil. A golden elixir that's full of flavor and nutrients, olive oil is truly the secret to the Mediterranean passion for cooking nutritious foods that taste great. Not to mention the fact that olive oil may be a key factor in protecting against heart disease.

In the fat-phobic 1990s, nutritionists in the United States often recommended a low-fat diet for heart patients. Today the recommendations have reversed because we now know that "good" fats are vital for pleasing the palate and taming inflammation in the arteries. It's not how much fat, but *what kind* that makes all the difference. Case in point: In the 1950s and 1960s, inhabitants of the Greek island of Crete had an unusually high fat intake—at least 40 percent of total calories—primarily in the form of olive oil.[1] Butter and other animal fats or hydrogenated fats were virtually unknown in the southern Mediterranean region at that time. Add to this the islanders' low intake of saturated-fat-rich meat, modest amounts of dairy (flavorful cheeses and yogurt), and the almost exclusive use of monounsaturated fat in the form of olive oil and you have a vivid account of how this population maintained such a low rate of heart disease.[2] Sadly, with the demise of the traditional Mediterranean lifestyle and the move toward Western dietary and inactivity habits, disease rates in this region have climbed exponentially.

WHAT IS OLIVE OIL?

Olive oil is actually a fruit juice because it is made from crushing and pressing a whole fruit (olive)—pits and all—as opposed to a seed (such as rapeseed, the source of canola oil) or a vegetable (corn). In fact, it is the most widely consumed "fruit juice" in the world. Because olives are a fruit, they provide a large amount of plant antioxidants called polyphenols, which are scarce in other oils derived from seeds or vegetables. The minimal processing of extra virgin olive oil makes for a healthier fat because of the more natural state of the plant oil and the lack of excess heat and chemicals used to process it. Moreover, olive oil is one of the few oils that retain the natural flavor, antioxidants, vitamins, minerals, and other healthful components of the vegetable or seed, or, in this instance, the ripe olive fruit.

ORIGIN OF OLIVE OIL

The olive *(Olea europaea)* is a tree crop native to the Mediterranean basin and therefore is well adapted to the region's poor soil, hilly terrain, and arid climate. Carbon dating at a site in Spain shows olive seeds found there to be eight thousand years old. For the more than 750 years that ancient Rome ruled the Mediterranean, wheat, barley, figs, olives, grapes, and various fruits and vegetables—most of the foods we associate with the traditional Mediterranean diet—were established as part of the diet because of great demand from the Roman people.[3] For these reasons olive oil became the principal source of fat in all Mediterranean-style diets and for centuries has remained a staple in the Mediterranean style of eating. Currently, about 95 percent of the world's olive trees are located in the Mediterranean countries.

HEALTH BENEFITS OF THE KING OF FATS

Hippocrates called olive oil "the great therapeutic." Homer referred to it as "liquid gold." Olive oil's myriad health benefits can be attributed to three key compounds: monounsaturated fat (oleic acid), polyphenol antioxidant compounds, and the antioxidant vitamin E. So let's take a closer look at each of these miraculous olive oil ingredients.

Monounsaturated fat

Olive oil is made up of triglycerides that contain a large percentage of monounsaturated fatty acids. Up to 80 percent of olive oil is monounsaturated, primarily the omega-9 fatty acid known as oleic acid. The high monounsaturated fatty acid content of olive oil is extremely cardioprotective—it cuts your "bad" LDL cholesterol level, helps stabilize vulnerable plaque by preventing LDL from becoming oxidized (a key step in perpetuating atherosclerosis), and can bump up your level of HDL, the "good" cholesterol.[4] In fact, the monounsaturated fatty acids in olive oil are more effective in raising HDL than the polyunsaturated fatty acids found in high concentrations in vegetable oils.[5] Clearly, olive oil should be a staple in any diet geared toward treating and reversing heart disease.

OLIVE OIL AS SOLE FAT SLASHES HEART ATTACK RISK

A study out of Greece compared 700 men and 148 women with diagnosed heart disease to a similar group of healthy people. Results from the Cardio2000 study found that even when researchers adjusted for other variables such as smoking and high blood pressure, subjects who used olive oil exclusively cut their risk of having a heart attack by 49 percent compared to those who rarely consumed olive oil. (Consuming other types of fats and/or oils provided no protection.)

A similar study out of Spain compared the diets of 171 patients hospitalized with a recent heart attack with age-matched controls. This time, results showed that patients consuming the greatest amount of olive oil (approximately 3 tablespoons per day) had a whopping 82 percent reduced risk of a heart attack compared to those who rarely consumed olive oil.

The message? A habitual high intake of extra virgin olive oil—used as your primary source of fat—will provide you with a continual supply of potent disease-fighting antioxidants and oxidation-resistant fat, which can mediate and reverse plaque buildup in your arteries and cut your risk of a second heart attack by at least half and maybe more.

Sources: M. D. Kontogianni et al., "The impact of olive oil consumption pattern on the risk of acute coronary syndromes: The Cardio2000 case-control study," *Clinical Cardiology* 30 (2007): 125–129; and E. Fernández-Jarne et al., "Risk of first non-fatal myocardial infarction negatively associated with olive oil consumption: A case-control study in Spain," *International Journal of Epidemiology* 31, no. 2 (2002): 474–480.

Olive oil is not the only food rich in monounsaturated fat. Both avocado and almonds contain a nice quantity of this "good" fat, so add these foods to your diet too. Although in the kitchen many people think of avocados as a vegetable, botanically speaking, they are a fruit—and what a fruit! Avocados are loaded with potassium, a mineral that combats high blood pressure, antioxidant vitamins C and E, and bioactive phytochemicals as well as folate and fiber. Try spreading avocado on your sandwich as a delicious and healthful alternative to saturated-fat-laden mayonnaise.

Polyphenols

Phytochemicals is the term used to describe the thousands of nutrients found in edible plants that play a major role in preventing, halting, and reversing the process of atherosclerosis. Phytochemicals (*phyto-* comes from the Greek word for "plant") are found in fruits, vegetables, grains, and other plant foods. Polyphenols are the largest and most biologically active group of phytochemicals and the most abundant antioxidants in the diet. Polyphenols carry extraordinarily salutary effects, especially for the heart. Plants produce polyphenols to protect themselves against the elements: ultraviolet (UV) light damage and invasion by bacteria, fungi, and viruses. Polyphenols are therefore how the plants respond to stress damage and are what they use to heal themselves, in effect, natural antibiotics. As you probably guessed, certain types of olive oil contain an abundance of health-promoting phytochemicals, especially the major class of phytochemicals, the spectacular polyphenols.

EXTRA VIRGIN, EXTRA PHENOLS, EXTRA HEALTH

When surveying the crowded oil section of your supermarket aisle, note that there *is* a difference between "olive oil," "refined olive oil," "pure olive oil," "pomace olive oil," "virgin olive oil," and "extra virgin olive oil." Olive oil comes in different grades, with quality standards set by the International Olive Oil Council (IOOC). Make sure to choose a bottle with the words *extra virgin*. Extra virgin is the label awarded by the IOOC to only the purest and best of olive oils, those obtained from the first pressing of the olives and containing an acidity level below 0.8 percent (less than 0.8 grams of free oleic acid per 100 grams of oil). Plus, the oil must have been extracted mechanically without the use of excess heat or chemicals.

Italian scientists set out to prove that to obtain maximum heart health benefits, it really does matter what type of oil you ingest. In their study involving twelve healthy men, the researchers administered subjects one of three varieties of oil: extra virgin olive oil (polyphenol rich), virgin olive oil (negligible polyphenols), or corn oil (devoid of polyphenols), then proceeded to analyze the men's blood, measuring markers of inflammation and oxidative stress.[6] The results came back loud and clear: Extra virgin olive oil was the *only fat* that tamed inflammation and raised the antioxidant capacity of the subjects' blood. This is because the phenol compounds are lost in the processing of other grades of olive oils and because there are no antioxidant polyphenols at all in corn oil.

And what's so great about those polyphenols? The most abundant polyphenols in olive oil, hydroxytyrosol and oleuropein, are particularly useful in the treatment of heart disease because they can be absorbed by the LDL cholesterol particle, further increasing its resistance to oxidation (the process that instigates plaque formation in the arteries). Another advantage of these special olive oil antioxidants is that they contribute to taming oxidative stress, the physiological state that promotes inflammation and plaque growth right where it counts, *inside* the inner wall of your arteries. Olive oil antioxidants can disarm those damaging free radical molecules, the ones that perpetuate the process of atherosclerosis and are hidden within the subterranean intima—the spot where plaque buildup occurs—as opposed to other types of antioxidants, which are restricted to scavenging free radicals circulating in the bloodstream.[7] You should know that oxidative stress must be tempered to effectively reverse your disease. So what exactly is oxidative stress? It is an imbalance between free radical production and your body's internal antioxidant capacity. Free radicals form as a by-product of normal metabolism and through environmental factors such as X-rays, UV light, and pollution. The best strategy for controlling free radical formation, thereby slowing and reversing plaque buildup, is to maintain a balance between oxidants and antioxidants— promoting an optimal physiological state. Consuming extra virgin olive oil (EVOO) is one daily medication you should take to tip this balance in your heart's favor. Hence, this ability of olive oil polyphenols to obstruct oxidation of plaque-building components deep within the arterial wall is akin to a firefighter pouring water on flames—it calms the inflammation, which is key to reversing atherosclerosis.

GO SPANISH FOR MAXIMUM ANTIOXIDANT POWER

If your supermarket carries extra virgin olive oil that has been derived from the Picual variety of olives, purchase that one. One study has shown that the Picual variety demonstrates an unusually high antioxidant activity. Picual olive oils come from Jaén province in the south of Spain, representing approximately 25 percent of the world's olive oil production. In fact, Spain is the top producer and exporter of olive oil, with close to five million acres of olive trees. The darker varieties also are a better choice, because black olives have a much greater concentration of antioxidant phenolic compounds than green olives. But don't pour on the tasty antioxidant-rich olive oil with complete abandon or you will pay at the scale . . . olive oil, just like all other fats and oils, still adds 120 calories per tablespoon to your total daily calorie count.

Sources: C. Samaniego Sánchez et al., "Different radical scavenging tests in virgin olive oil and their relation to the total phenol content," *Analytica Chimica Acta* 593, no. 1 (2007): 103–107; and R. W Owen et al., "Olives and olive oil in cancer prevention," *European Journal of Cancer Prevention* 13 (2004): 319–326.

Vitamin E

Extra virgin olive oil is an excellent food source of vitamin E, a major dietary antioxidant vitamin. Getting in your daily dose of olive oil will elevate the level of vitamin E circulating in your bloodstream. This is important, because low levels of vitamin E in the blood are associated with a significantly higher frequency of heart disease as well as increased occurrence of *stenotic* plaque (the hard, thick, calcium-filled plaque that tends to clog the coronary arteries).[8] Because vitamin E is fat soluble, it also incorporates into the LDL cholesterol particle, offering your LDL cholesterol particles another avenue of protection against free radical attack. Vitamin E can retard the development and progression of atherosclerosis not only by protecting LDL from oxidation but also with its unique ability to stifle arterial smooth muscle cells from multiplying and contributing to plaque formation. (Recall from Chapter 2 that smooth muscle cells play a large role in providing the structure of plaque and in the evolution of the innocuous fatty streak to the dangerous type of rupture-prone vulnerable plaque.)

FDA HEALTH CLAIM FOR OLIVE OIL

So strong is the science supporting the cardioprotective effect of consuming olive oil that in 2004 the U.S. Food and Drug Administration (FDA) issued a qualified health claim for olive oil that reads something like this: There is limited but not conclusive evidence suggesting that consuming about two tablespoons (23 grams) of olive oil a day may reduce the risk of coronary heart disease because of the monounsaturated fat in olive oil.[9] (*Note:* We have since learned that the health benefits of olive oil stem from much more than just the monounsaturated fat content.)

One additional advantage of using olive oil in the kitchen is that it is loaded with flavor and encourages the consumption of large amounts of vegetables and legumes—antioxidant and fiber-rich foods that many Americans find difficult to fit into their diet.

Because it is unclear whether it is the olive oil alone or that the notable health benefits are associated with a combination of olive oil and vegetables, legumes, and fish, you would be wise to make olive oil your main fat and use it liberally in combination with the other foods outlined in this book. In salads or in cooking, the exquisite taste of olive oil can complement any dish. Add in flavorful herbs and spices and you have an antioxidant powerhouse that will bring to life the Mediterranean way of eating, rich in grains, legumes, vegetables, and fruits and a generous amount of liquid gold—extra virgin olive oil.

DAILY HEART DISEASE REVERSAL STRATEGY: OLIVE OIL'S CONTRIBUTION

Strategy 1. Boost total antioxidant capacity

Consuming your daily dose of extra virgin olive oil will contribute to raising your body's total antioxidant capacity (TAC), the primary means by which your body fights off harmful free radicals. Free radicals wreak havoc in the body, enabling LDL cholesterol to fuel inflammation, plaque growth, and atherosclerosis. Olive oil is a simple and surefire way to increase TAC and combat free radicals—and research proves it's quick, as it takes only two hours for a person's total antioxidant capacity to escalate after consuming extra virgin olive oil.[10]

Some other scientifically proven strategies for raising your TAC:

1. Consume a large range of antioxidants in the foods you eat throughout the day, such as those containing powerful, plant-derived polyphenols (like extra virgin olive oil), along with food-derived antioxidant vitamins E and C and provitamin A. These antioxidants are all potent anti-inflammatory agents.

2. Perform a daily bout of antioxidant-boosting exercise.

Disease reversal works via consistently maintaining a high level of antioxidants in your bloodstream, because your ability to scavenge free radicals is the first line of defense against artery-damaging oxidative stress. Hence, the Prevent a Second Heart Attack plan is designed to *maximize your total antioxidant capacity* on any given day by having you consume the wide spectrum of antioxidant-rich foods recommended in this book—including olive oil—and perform the exercise that stimulates your body's production of natural antioxidant enzymes.

Strategy 2. Immunize LDL against free radical attack

Consuming your daily dose of extra virgin olive oil will supply your body with both monounsaturated fatty acids and antioxidants. These two olive oil components each protect the LDL particle (although in different ways).

Monounsaturated fat has a stable molecular structure and when it incorporates into the wall of LDL cholesterol, it strengthens it against oxidation, ultimately thwarting plaque formation. Polyunsaturated fat, in contrast, is weaker and prone to oxidation, especially the omega-6 type of polyunsaturated fat discussed in depth in Chapter 10. Excess consumption of certain types of polyunsaturated fat can contribute to the plaque-building process—hence this is the primary reason why you should make stable monounsaturated-rich EVOO your main fat. The antioxidant phenols (including vitamin E) in extra virgin olive oil work hand in hand with monounsaturated fat to protect the LDL particles by scavenging free radicals *inside* the arterial wall (intima), which is where LDL oxidation occurs.

Strategy 3. Control cholesterol

Consuming your daily dose of extra virgin olive oil provides a dual benefit—it both raises good HDL cholesterol and lowers bad LDL. (Remember, you want to try to achieve those "ideal" cholesterol levels discussed in Chapter 1: LDL less than 70 mg/dL and HDL greater than 60 mg/dL.) But it also has a third benefit: Extra virgin olive oil can actually increase the *size* of LDL particles— enlarging them so they are less likely to pierce the arterial wall and become oxidized.[11] Recall that small and heavy LDL particles are the dangerous kind because they accelerate the development of atherosclerosis. Change their shape and you take an additional step in fighting your disease.

HDL cholesterol particles are the garbage trucks that scoop up cholesterol from the arterial wall and drop it off at the liver, where it is excreted. Hence, the higher your HDL value, the better. Relatively few foods have a major impact on raising your HDL, but thankfully, olive oil is one of them. Once again, go for the extra virgin olive oil to get maximum cholesterol benefits—studies show that EVOO has a much greater HDL-boosting effect than refined olive oil.

Strategy 4. Fight inflammation

Consuming your daily dose of extra virgin olive oil will soothe inflammation of your arteries by stimulating your cells' production of anti-inflammatory agents.[12] When your arteries' endothelial cells are exposed to LDL particles enriched with oleic acid (the monounsaturated fat in olive oil), they sprout fewer adhesion molecules—those sticky Velcro-like molecules that attract white blood cells and grow from endothelial cells once they become "activated." By making the walls of your arteries less sticky, olive oil effectively nips inflammation in the bud. The olive oil–enriched LDL particles no longer tell white blood cells to stick to the endothelium, and the phenols in the olive oil itself thwart endothelium activation, making olive oil a fantastic remedy for inflammation.

One ingredient of olive oil that we haven't discussed is oleocanthal, which has been discovered and isolated only recently. What's interesting about oleocanthal is that scientists discovered that it relieves pain and lowers inflammation to the same degree as the familiar over-the-counter anti-inflammatory medication ibuprofen (Motrin or Advil).[13] So forget about aspirin; EVOO is the new wonder drug for this millennium!

Strategy 5. Lower blood pressure

If I haven't yet convinced you of olive oil's miraculous powers, here's one more benefit to add to the list: Consuming your daily dose of extra virgin olive oil will lower your blood pressure.

But how? Olive oil contains two ingredients that dampen the squeeze on your blood vessels. Scientists believe that olive oil's blood-pressure-lowering action is highly related to the "good," heart-healthy monounsaturated fat (oleic acid) content of olive oil.[14] The propensity for oleic acid to incorporate into the cell membranes of arteries changes the cells' physiology—reducing the amount of a certain protein in cells that promotes constriction of blood vessels. Reduce the amount of the protein that squeezes the vessels, and you automatically relax them and blood pressure drops. In the body, oleic acid also lowers blood pressure via another route. It is transformed into the other kind of heart-healthy, good fat, omega-3. The olive oil–derived omega-3 fatty acid is called trienoic acid, which also has a relaxing effect on the arteries—causing them to dilate and thereby reduce blood pressure.[15]

High blood pressure is a great concern for people with heart disease, because it is related to dysfunction of the endothelium, hence contributing to instability of plaque and the likelihood of a second cardiac event. You *must* control your blood pressure to protect against a second heart attack. Consuming extra virgin olive oil is an excellent (and tasty) complement to your blood pressure medication in helping you achieve this goal.

Strategy 6. Improve blood sugar; prevent and treat diabetes

Consuming extra virgin olive oil daily will also help prevent and treat diabetes. People with diabetes, especially uncontrolled diabetes, are at great risk for plaque buildup, because the extra sugar in the bloodstream fuels endothelial dysfunction and plaque growth. (As noted previously, most people with diabetes will die of heart disease.)

The monounsaturated fat found in olive oil helps lower the insulin requirement (via improved insulin sensitivity) of people with diabetes, and it even improves glucose metabolism in healthy individuals.[16] Any way you look at it, olive oil is good medicine for stabilizing blood sugar and for preventing and treating this dangerous disease.

OLIVE OIL CUTS BLOOD PRESSURE, REDUCES MEDICATION DOSAGE

An Italian study found that administering a daily dose of olive oil to people previously diagnosed with high blood pressure not only lowered their pressure but also allowed them to reduce their medication dosage. Twenty-three people with diagnosed high blood pressure were administered either sunflower oil or olive oil in addition to their usual diet (three to four "spoonfuls" of oil per day) over six months. Only the olive oil group showed a significant reduction in blood pressure and daily blood pressure drug requirement (in fact, eight subjects in the olive oil group were able to go off their blood pressure medication entirely). The authors stated that this phenomenon occurred because of the ability of olive oil polyphenols to stimulate endothelial cells' production of nitric oxide—the substance that causes arteries to relax and dilate—thereby reducing blood pressure and easing inflammation.

Source: L. Aldo Ferrara et al., "Olive oil and reduced need for antihypertensive medication," *Archives of Internal Medicine* 160 (2000): 837–842.

Strategy 7. Promote an anti-clotting milieu in the blood

Additionally, incorporating extra virgin olive oil into your diet will render the blood less likely to clot by interfering with the ability of platelets to stick to one another.[17] This is important because blood platelets stimulate growth of plaque by adhering to the endothelial layer of the arterial wall (refer to Chapter 2); therefore, platelets are a participant in vulnerable plaque remodeling. Furthermore, recall from Chapter 2 that heart attacks are most often caused by a blood clot sealing off the artery once a vulnerable plaque has ruptured. Thin the blood and you lessen your chances of either of these scenarios occurring.

Italian researchers at the University of Milan studied an extract of the olive oil antioxidant polyphenol hydroxytyrosol in their lab and found that the olive oil phenol extract completely inhibited blood platelets' ability to stick together and form a clot.[18]

Strategy 8. Balance omega-6:omega-3 ratio

Using extra virgin olive oil instead of other oils will decrease your intake of omega-6 fat and, more specifically, your intake of a polyunsaturated fatty acid called linoleic acid (LA). LA is ubiquitous in the foods typically consumed in the Western diet. It is the main fat in vegetable oils such as corn oil, safflower oil, and sunflower oil. The problem is that LA accounts for 90 percent of the fatty acids in the LDL particle—and because it is polyunsaturated, it is highly susceptible to free radical attack and oxidation, making LA a pro-inflammatory food.[19] Replacing oils loaded with LA with extra virgin olive oil will ultimately help you balance your omega-6:omega-3 ratio (more on this later), as well as generate oxidation-resistant LDL particles—thereby blocking inflammation and fighting the progression of heart disease.

TIPS FOR GETTING IN YOUR DAILY DOSE OF OLIVE OIL

• Keep a small opaque bottle of extra virgin olive oil on your kitchen counter (and the rest in a sealed, airtight metal tin in the refrigerator). Grab the bottle and use it for any and all types of cooking. Refill the small bottle on a weekly basis from the refrigerated container and let it warm to room temperature before using.

- Eat salads at lunch and dinner and dress with an easy-to-make and always delicious olive oil vinaigrette. Mix three parts olive oil with one part balsamic vinegar (another antioxidant-rich food), lemon juice, herbs, and a touch of Dijon mustard (see Chapter 16 for the specifics on preparing a quick, healthy, and delicious olive oil vinaigrette seasoned with fresh herbs).

- Pour a liberal amount of olive oil on fish before grilling.

- Coat vegetables generously before roasting or grilling.

- Drizzle olive oil over your plant foods to enhance their flavor: potatoes, bean soups, grains, and steamed vegetables.

- Routinely fill a small dish with a flavorful olive oil to use for dipping whole-wheat breads and other foods.

- Cut the top off an entire head of garlic, drizzle generously with olive oil, wrap in tinfoil, and bake—then use it as a spread for a crusty piece of whole-grain bread.

- Open a can of cannellini beans, rinse thoroughly, and purée with olive oil and garlic; season and serve as a dip.

THE FATS OF LIFE: MAKE YOURS OLIVE OIL

In the end, it is not the amount of fat in the diet that dictates the health of your arteries, but the type. In the countries that border the Mediterranean, people have historically consumed a high-fat diet, yet their rates of chronic disease are exceptionally low. But where are they getting all this "good fat"? They harvest it from the fruits of Mother Nature's splendid gift to humankind, the truly life-giving olive tree.

Extra virgin olive oil is unique and superior to all other fat for two distinct reasons. It contains a large concentration of heart-protective monounsaturated fat as well as a remarkable amount of disease-fighting antioxidants—the only fat that contains this high a level of antioxidant potency. The synergy between the monounsaturated fatty acids and phytochemicals makes olive oil truly a super food for the heart and king of all fats. So be sure to take in a good daily dose of extra virgin olive oil on your salads, fish, vegetables, and pasta and its delicate taste will surely satisfy your taste buds as well as soothe your arteries.

Heart-Healthy Food Number 2: Greens and Other Vegetables

We are indeed much more than what we eat, but what we eat can
nevertheless help us to be much more than what we are.

—Adelle Davis, pioneer nutritionist and author (1904–1974)

 Eat a dark green leafy salad at least once daily.

Companion foods Rx: at least five additional colorful vegetables, including one cruciferous, every day

Primary disease-fighting bioactive compounds:

- Polyphenols such as the flavonoids, especially flavonols (quercetin)
  and anthocyanins
- Carotenoids such as lutein and zeaxanthin
- Organosulfur compounds such as indoles
- Vitamins (especially antioxidants: vitamin C, beta-carotene, and
  vitamin E)

VERDURE: THE LEADING LADY

Think simple and make your first course a salad dressed with olive oil and fresh lemon juice or wine vinegar. Although Mediterranean food customs differ somewhat, the term *salad* generally means a symphony of green leaves.

The foundation of Mediterranean cuisine is built around vegetables. If you want to harness the power of antioxidants to fight atherosclerosis, you need to eat plants—and lots of them. Plant foods have the ability to prevent illness and heal, especially deep, dark greens drenched in olive oil—heart and blood pressure medicine, Mediterranean style—taken on a daily basis.

Ancel Keys, the American physiologist and founder of the "Mediterranean diet" concept, described the plethora of green leafy vegetables at the heart of the Mediterranean eating style simply as "leaves," or *verdure*: "No main meal in the Mediterranean countries is replete without lots of *verdure* (greens)," he

---

HEART ATTACK PREVENTION SUPERFOOD: SPINACH

Everyone knows Popeye got his megamuscles from downing those cans of spinach, but what you may not know is that his heart was as strong as his biceps. This is because calorie for calorie, spinach is one of the most nutrient-dense foods on earth. Spinach is exceptionally rich in flavonols (namely, quercetin) and has a very high antioxidant activity, according to the Oxygen Radical Absorbance Capacity (ORAC) scale—the most common laboratory method of assessing the antioxidant capacity of various foods.

Sources: Anna R. Proteggente et al., "The antioxidant activity of regularly consumed fruit and vegetables reflects their phenolic and vitamin C composition," *Free Radical Research* 36, no. 2 (2002): 217–233; and Guohua Cao et al., "Serum antioxidant capacity is increased by consumption of strawberries, spinach, red wine, or vitamin C in elderly women," *Journal of Nutrition* 128 (1998): 2383–2390.

wrote in 1995.[1] Just how much *verdure* should you be eating? The traditional Mediterranean diet includes a huge consumption of vegetables, corresponding to about 4 cups per day *in addition to* about 3 cups of "wild greens," which refers to a plant called purslane.[2] Purslane is actually a highly nutritious trailing plant and common weed that thrives in dry conditions, and hence it grows well along the arid coastline of Crete. It is packed with vitamin C, phytochemicals, and a small amount of the hard-to-find but exceptionally heart-healthy omega-3 fat alpha-linolenic acid (ALA). Because purslane is not generally commercially available in the United States—although it does grow just about everywhere and could easily be harvested—substituting dark leafy greens such as spinach and arugula for your daily dose of greens is a practical strategy for filling this Prevent a Second Heart Attack daily food prescription.

THE COLOR OF HEALTH

Fresh, colorful vegetables: dark green and leafy; red, ripe, and juicy; or bright orange and crunchy. This exquisite rainbow-colored cornucopia is truly the class of foods that keeps our arteries healthy and clean. Head for your greengrocer and harness the phenomenal medicinal power of natural plant compounds. Buy them fresh, buy them often, and fill your body with a spectrum of healthy colors, nature's medicine chest. Greeks consume an average of nine servings of antioxidant-rich fruits and vegetables a day. It takes the typical American *three days* to eat that much!

Use the following chart to help you make the best vegetable choices on a daily basis. And be sure to add some color to your plate *throughout* the day, not just crammed into one meal, to make sure your arteries have a continual supply of anti-inflammatory, antioxidant phytonutrients.

Color-Code Your Vegetables

Vegetable	Daily Serving	Sample Foods	Primary Antioxidants
Dark leafy greens and cruciferous vegetables	At least one	Spinach, dark green varieties of lettuce, collard greens,* mustard greens,* romaine, broccoli,* cabbage,* cauliflower,* rutabaga,* turnips,* kale,* Brussels sprouts,* oriental cabbage,* arugula,* watercress,* radish,* daikon,* wasabi,* bok choy*	Carotenoids *(lutein, zeaxanthin, beta-carotene);* flavonoids *(quercetin, kaempferol, myricetin);* organosulfur compounds* *(indoles, isothiocyanates)*
Red/purple vegetables	At least one	Beets, ketchup, salsa, cooked tomato products (such as tomato sauce), tomatoes, sun-dried tomatoes, low-sodium vegetable juice, eggplant, red pepper, red onion, radicchio	Carotenoids *(lycopene);* flavonoids *(anthocyanins)*
Yellow/orange vegetables	At least one	Carrots, peppers (orange, yellow), pumpkin, winter squash, corn, sweet potatoes, yellow tomatoes	Carotenoids *(beta-carotene, beta-cryptoxanthin, lycopene)*
Green herbs	Use liberally, at least once	Basil, bay leaves, cilantro, dill weed, marjoram, mint, oregano, parsley, rosemary, sage, tarragon, thyme	Flavonoids *(apigenin, luteolin, quercetin);* phenolic acids *(rosemarinic acid, caffeic acid)*
Allium vegetables	Use liberally, at least once	Garlic, onions, green onions (chives), shallots, leeks	Organosulfur compounds *(allicin);* flavonoids *(quercetin, kaempferol, myricetin)*
Other vegetables	At least one	Artichoke, asparagus, celery, cucumber, green beans, green peppers, mushrooms, okra, parsnips, potatoes, snow peas, water chestnuts, zucchini	Flavonoids *(quercetin, kaempferol, myricetin)*

*Cruciferous vegetables.

Phytochemicals: Weapons against free-radical destruction

What makes vegetables so healthful? A major component is their high concentration of phytochemicals, a small army of disease-fighting agents, which are separate from—and potentially more valuable than—better-known vitamins and minerals. As you learned in Chapter 5, plants are virtual chemical factories and their "phyto" (plant) nutrients protect us against heart disease and premature aging.

More than eight thousand phytochemicals have been identified that are biologically active in humans and promote health; however, scientists believe that a large percentage remains to be discovered.[3] Researchers have developed a means of categorizing these plant chemicals based on the similarity of chemical structure. But don't let the scientific names intimidate you; they are simply a means of enabling us to identify which chemicals are concentrated

---

LOTS OF VEGGIES BOOST LONGEVITY

It is well known that the Mediterranean diet is best for extending life. To determine which components of the Mediterranean diet have the greatest effect on longevity, scientists recently analyzed data from the Greek segment (more than 23,000 healthy men and women) of the much larger-scale European Prospective Investigation into Cancer and Nutrition (EPIC) study. After an average of 8.5 years of follow-up, the researchers found that longevity was most associated with the following, in descending order of significance:

1. Moderate consumption of alcohol (red wine drunk with meals)
2. Low consumption of meat
3. High consumption of vegetables
4. High consumption of fruit and nuts
5. High consumption of olive oil
6. High consumption of legumes

The authors declared that when a high vegetable intake, moderate wine intake, and low meat consumption *are removed* from the traditional Mediterranean diet, the longevity benefits all but disappear.

Source: Antonia Trichopoulou, Christina Bamia, and Dimitrios Trichopoulos, "Anatomy of health effects of Mediterranean diet: Greek EPIC prospective cohort study," *British Medical Journal* 338 (2009): doi:10.1136/bmj.b2337.

in which foods. Some plant chemicals play a more protective role in heart disease than others (take flavonoids, for instance), so the classification system allows us to pinpoint the foods highest in these super-heart-healthy nutrients. When phytochemicals are consumed, their antioxidant and anti-inflammatory properties work in concert to mop up free radicals—the dangerous molecules that propagate inflammation. But don't be fooled by what supplement companies tell you—taking dietary supplements consisting of isolated pure antioxidant plant compounds does not have the same health-promoting effects as eating a plant-based diet. When taken in supplement form, the compounds lose their bioactivity or behave in different ways in the body and in some cases may even accelerate disease.[4]

DAILY HEART DISEASE REVERSAL STRATEGY: VEGETABLES' CONTRIBUTION

Strategy 1. Boost total antioxidant capacity and curtail inflammation

Consuming greens and other colorful vegetables contributes to raising your body's total antioxidant capacity (TAC). Recall from Chapter 5 that the best strategy for curbing plaque-building oxidative stress is to maintain a positive balance between antioxidants and pro-oxidants in your body. Providing your body with a steady stream of various dietary antioxidants—in other words, boosting your TAC over the course of the day—will give you the edge by preventing or slowing disease-causing oxidative stress and continuously dousing the inflammation that fuels your disease process.

Richest source of dietary antioxidants: polyphenols. Vegetables are chock-full of myriad polyphenols (the major disease-battling phytochemical), so let's take a closer look at the miraculous healing

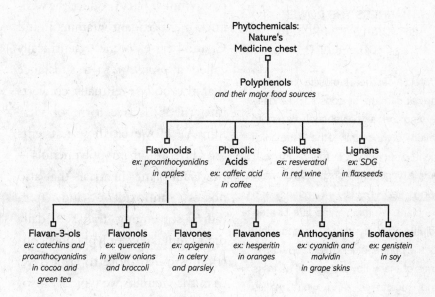

Figure 6.1. *Polyphenols* is the term used to describe a major class of bioactive phyto-chemicals scientifically proven to protect against heart disease. There are four main sub-classes of polyphenols: flavonoids, phenolic acids, stilbenes, and lignans.

power of plants. There are four main subclasses of polyphenols (Figure 6.1): flavonoids, phenolic acids, stilbenes, and lignans. Flavonoids account for about two thirds of our polyphenol intake, and phenolic acids for the remaining one third, with stilbenes and lignans accounting for just a small fraction of our total intake. Vegetables contain an abundance of flavonoids, the subclass of polyphenols that has garnered the most attention for its role in pre-venting and treating heart disease. There are six major subclasses of flavonoids: flavonols, flavones, isoflavones, flavanones, flavan-3-ols, and anthocyanins.

Polyphenols pack more antioxidant punch than vitamins. Plants are virtual chemical factories that churn out thousands of medicinal-like

HARNESS THE POWER OF PURPLE TO PROTECT YOUR HEART

Protect your heart muscle from free radical damage by consuming a daily serving of a polyphenol flavonoid called anthocyanin—the blue pigmented polyphenol found in red/purple vegetables such as red cabbage, red beets, radicchio, and eggplant. Anthocyanins are water-soluble pigments that are responsible for the purple, blue, violet, and mauve hues of many flowers as well as fruits and vegetables. And what makes purple veggies so heart-healthy? Anthocyanins provide cardioprotection by increasing the heart's production of glutathione, the primary antioxidant in heart cells.

Source: Marie-Claire Toufektsian et al., "Chronic dietary intake of plant-derived anthocyanins protects the rat heart against ischemia-reperfusion injury," Journal of Nutrition 138 (2008): 747–752.

compounds. They produce the well-known antioxidant vitamins E and C, and beta-carotene (scientifically called a *provitamin,* a substance that the body eventually converts into the bioactive form or vitamin A). However, these nutrients are different from polyphenols—powerful plant chemicals that also possess antioxidant and free-radical-scavenging traits. A daily dietary intake of polyphenols contributes much more to your TAC than the vitamins we typically associate with antioxidant protection.

Let's draw a comparison to a familiar antioxidant vitamin, vitamin C. Although vitamin C is an extremely valuable water-soluble antioxidant, its disease-fighting strength pales in comparison to polyphenols. That is because we consume so much more—ten times the amount of polyphenols compared to vitamin C. One study demonstrated that the catechin polyphenol called epigallocatechin gallate (EGCG)—found in high concentration in green tea—has twenty times the antioxidant power of vitamin C.[5] In fact, more than 80 percent of the TAC from vegetables comes from bioactive phytochemicals other than vitamin C.[6]

That's not to say that antioxidant vitamins are not important in the fight against heart disease. The body's antioxidant defense system is complex, incorporating both "fast-acting" antioxidants such as vitamin C and "slow-acting" antioxidants such as polyphenols.[7]

All types of dietary antioxidants counteract the many types of free radicals generated in the body, and each makes a valuable contribution to your TAC. This integrated action from numerous compounds is why a wide variety of antioxidant-rich foods should be consumed on a daily basis.[8]

Help put out the arterial fire with organosulfur compounds. Using copious amounts of garlic and onions to flavor your food can also lessen inflammation in the arteries, and of course no Mediterranean meal would be complete without garlic and onions. Garlic and onions fall under a different class of phytochemicals than the polyphenols. They are known as organosulfur compounds, as are the cruciferous veggies (ultra-healthy heart disease and cancer-prevention vegetables such as broccoli and cauliflower). Foods rich in organosulfur compounds are recognizable by their characteristic pungent odor and flavor. Garlic boosts the immune system by stimulating the activity of our body's main defense weapon—natural killer T cells.[9] What's more, garlic can modestly lower "bad" LDL cholesterol as well as thin the blood, making platelets less able to bond together to form clots. Onions are also considered natural anticlotting agents, because they too possess substances that interfere with platelets' ability to stick together.

Add carotenoids to your anti-inflammatory arsenal. Carotenoids are fat-soluble plant pigments that give flowers and plants some of their most vibrant colors. As with other types of phytochemicals, dietary carotenoids inhibit the onset and proliferation of heart disease by virtue of their strong antioxidant properties. They are also potent anti-inflammatory compounds that boost immune system function,[10] and they fight off arterial irritation using different types of biological actions than other dietary antioxidants.[11]

There are several subclasses of carotenoids with names you may be familiar with, such as beta-carotene, lutein, and lycopene (Figure 6.2).

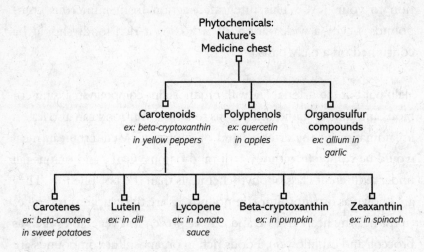

Figure 6.2. Carotenoids are a class of phytochemicals that differ from polyphenols. They are fat-soluble plant pigments responsible for the bright red, yellow, and orange hues of fruits and vegetables. Carotenoids exert potent anti-inflammatory action.

Beta-carotene gives carrots their vivid orange color. Beta-carotene is also one of the most important of these plant pigments because the body forms vitamin A from it. Vitamin A has many vital functions; it is necessary for maintaining the integrity of skin, hair, and other tissues as well as for proper immune system function and vision. Beta-carotene also affects the health of your arteries, because it scavenges free radicals deep within the LDL particle. Lycopene is another type of carotenoid or plant pigment that is important to include in your day as a warrior against plaque buildup. Lycopene gives vegetables such as tomatoes their red hue, and red is often good for the heart. To maximize lycopene's disease-fighting ability, make sure to eat cooked tomato products, such as

CAROTENOIDS: MIRACLE MEDICINE FOR
HEART DISEASE REVERSAL

Lutein and its companion carotenoids, zeaxanthin and beta-cryptoxanthin—pigments found in high concentration in dark leafy greens such as spinach and kale—are strong antioxidants that can protect against the progression of atherosclerosis. This is according to findings from the Los Angeles Atherosclerosis Study of 573 middle-aged men and women at the University of Southern California Keck School of Medicine. Ultrasound examination of the neck arteries of the subjects found that participants with high blood levels of three carotenoids (lutein, zeaxanthin, and beta-cryptoxanthin) exhibited significantly slowed progression of atherosclerosis.

Results of a Swedish study shed light on the effects of carotenoids and oxidation. Swedish scientists investigated why death from heart disease in 50- to 54-year-old men is four times higher in Lithuania than in Sweden. A striking finding was that even though the Lithuanian men had a *lower* level of bad LDL cholesterol, the LDL was very prone to oxidation. The Lithuanian men also had lower blood levels of the antioxidant carotenoids lycopene and beta-carotene. The researchers surmised that the high mortality rate from heart disease in Lithuania was not as related to the traditional risk factors such as high blood pressure and smoking, which were similar between the men, but instead was linked to the low carotenoid antioxidant state of the Lithuanians' blood and the consequential increase in LDL vulnerability to oxidation.

Australian researchers were curious which foods will give you the biggest carotenoid bang for your bite. They performed a study that pinpointed three carotenoid-rich foods that are staples in the Mediterranean diet: *dark green leafy vegetables, figs,* and *extra virgin olive oil.* It is no coincidence that these are three of the eight foods recommended in the Prevent a Second Heart Attack plan.

Sources: James H. Dwyer et al., "Progression of carotid intima-media thickness and plasma antioxidants: The Los Angeles Atherosclerosis Study," *Arteriosclerosis, Thrombosis, and Vascular Biology* 24 (2003): 313–319; Margareta Kritenson et al., "Antioxidant state and mortality from coronary heart disease in Lithuanian and Swedish men: Concomitant cross sectional study of men aged 50," *British Medical Journal* 314 (1997): 629–633; and Q. Su et al.,"Identification and quantification of major carotenoids in selected components of the Mediterranean diet: Green leafy vegetables, figs and olive oil," *European Journal of Clinical Nutrition* 56 (2002): 1149–1154.

tomato sauce, often. This is because the cooking process liberates the more biologically active form of lycopene.

Strategy 2. Prevent or treat diabetes

Consuming green leafy vegetables can slash your risk of developing diabetes, which, as you know, greatly accelerates atherosclerosis. A study of 71,346 healthy nurses followed over eighteen years and published in the journal *Diabetes Care* found that eating just one serving of dark leafy greens (including bok choy, cabbage, dark lettuces, kale, spinach, watercress, and mustard greens) per day cuts the risk of developing type 2 diabetes. Each additional daily serving of dark greens the nurses ate led to a 9 percent drop in the risk of diabetes.[12] What's more, carotenoids (spinach is loaded with carotenoids) can halve your risk of contracting metabolic syndrome—a condition characterized by belly fat accumulation and insulin resistance that often leads to diabetes and accelerates plaque buildup. A recent Dutch study of 374 men age forty to eighty showed that men reporting higher carotenoid intakes (mainly beta-carotene and lycopene) were 58 percent less likely to have metabolic syndrome.[13]

Another good reason to eat your broccoli. Consistently high levels of blood sugar in people with "uncontrolled" diabetes raises the amount of free radicals generated at the level of the endothelium. *People with diabetes have a much higher level of free radicals circulating in their blood vessels than people without diabetes, particularly in vessels supplying organs most vulnerable to diabetic damage such as the eyes, kidneys, and heart.*[14] This situation results in excessive free radical damage to the fragile endothelial layer of the arterial walls and contributes to the dramatically elevated rates of death from heart disease in people with diabetes. So if you are diabetic, it is imperative that you get in your daily array of intensely colored, antioxidant-rich vegetables to treat or prevent this problem. (See "Color-Code Your Vegetables" on page 112.) Researchers have shown that one group of vegetables in particular, those in the *Bras-*

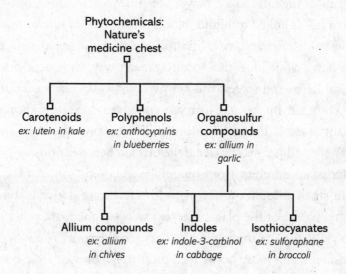

Figure 6.3. Eat cruciferous vegetables often to bathe your bloodstream in organosulfur compounds, nature's prescription for prevention of both heart disease and cancer.

sica genus (mustard family), are potential disease fighters. Vegetables with organosulfur compounds (a.k.a. the "anti-cancer" vegetables), which include cruciferous vegetables such as broccoli, Brussels sprouts, and cabbages (Figure 6.3), can effectively treat endothelial dysfunction and heart vessel damage in people with diabetes, and watercress can actually prevent free radical damage in the first place.[15]

FLAVOR YOUR LIFE WITH HERBS AND SPICES

We may not have reached the fish chapter of *Prevent a Second Heart Attack* yet, but you should dog-ear this page for when we do! Because as soon as you are ready to grill your fresh-off-the-boat halibut steak, you should be sure to season it with a little chopped fresh dill, some minced garlic, and a squeeze of lemon. If you've brought out the salt shaker, maybe it's time to reconsider. Salt—too much of it—is linked to higher blood pressure and premature death from heart disease, and we eat far too much of it in our diets. Learning to flavor your food the Mediterranean way, with delicious and healthful herbs and spices, will kill two birds with one stone: It will lower your salt intake and increase your heart-disease-fighting antioxidant arsenal. Using herbs and spices to flavor your foods can add variety and help you make delicious kitchen creations.

Herbs are different from vegetables in cooking in that they are used in small amounts to flavor food. Herbs are derived from the leafy green part of the plant, whereas spices come from other parts of the plant such as the seeds, the bark, or the root. You may want to consider using more herbs and spices to flavor your food because they possess legions of medicinal properties and, when eaten in conjunction with the healthy foods described in this book, will add to your plant power in fending off heart disease.

Herbs and spices such as dill, rosemary, oregano, onions, garlic, ginger, turmeric, cinnamon, and mustard offer you lots more than just flavor. They possess an extraordinary amount of active phytochemicals including carotenoids, polyphenols (especially the flavone subclass of flavonoids), other types of phenols (such as apriole, carvacrol, and rosemarinic acid), and indoles such as allicin. Scientists believe that herbs' ability to enhance immune system function is related to three components in particular: flavonoids, vitamin C, and carotenoids.[16]

A few easily found herbs deserve special mention. Capers, for example, are a common ingredient in Mediterranean cuisine. If you were to take a trip to the Greek islands, and if you knew what to look for, you would most likely notice a shrub growing along the walls of the rocks that tower over the sea. Capers are the small buds of this plant that have been pickled in salt and vinegar. They are intensely flavorful, so a very little goes a long way; hence you can avoid the sodium overload. These small buds pack a big antioxidant punch, according to a study from Italy.[17] A small extract of capers was found to have a significant antioxidant effect comparable to that of the heart-healthy antioxidant vitamin E. Capers contain a nice dose of rutin, a powerful antioxidant flavonoid that once again, if used to flavor your food, will contribute to building your daily antioxidant defense system. (Just be sure to give the capers a quick rinse before using to eliminate excess salt.)

Oregano is another example of an indispensable herb that permeates Mediterranean-style dishes. Used commonly in tomato sauce, on vegetables, or in combination with olive oil and lemon to give Greek salad its distinctive flavor, oregano is truly a powerhouse of antioxidant activity. Oregano contains numerous types of phytochemicals, such as the phenolic acids, rosemarinic acid, and caffeic acid, as well as the flavonoids quercetin and apigenin. The large amount of antioxidants in oregano gives it high marks on the ORAC scientific assay.

TIPS FOR GETTING IN YOUR DAILY DOSE OF VEGETABLES

• Routinely eat a dark green salad appetizer at lunch and dinner when eating in or out, and remember to dress it simply with extra virgin olive oil and wine vinegar and/or fresh lemon juice.

• For quick and healthy, try purchasing prewashed, bagged, and prechopped vegetables, toss them on a sheet of tinfoil, drizzle with extra virgin olive oil, and roast (425° F for at least 30 minutes). Keep them in a container in the refrigerator for easy access.

• Purchase frozen vegetables (with a short ingredients list). Frozen vegetables, picked and frozen immediately after harvest, are a nutritionally sound choice when you don't have time to prepare tastier fresh vegetables. (In fact, frozen spinach has been shown to retain its carotenoid power longer than fresh because of the lower temperatures at which it is stored.)

- If the weather's nice, fire up the grill and roast vegetables coated in extra virgin olive oil.

- Infuse fresh herbs into your olive oil or mix them into your salad dressing (olive oil vinaigrette) to add extra flavor and antioxidant power.

- When time doesn't allow for prepping fresh veggies, grab a bottle of jarred veggies, such as corn or roasted red peppers. Just watch out for added sodium, and if the veggies are packed in oil, check to ensure that it's olive oil.

- You can always get an array of colorful vegetables at a salad bar (some supermarkets even have them). Avoid the mayonnaise or oil-added veggie selections. Pile on the plain colorful vegetables instead and dress with olive oil and a splash of balsamic vinegar.

- Remember, no lunch or dinner without that rainbow of vegetables!

MOM WAS RIGHT: EAT YOUR GREENS!

Eating Italian doesn't mean a heaping plate of spaghetti and meatballs. On the contrary, the true Italian meal features a kaleidoscope of colors. Why not choose food fresh from the garden, beginning with a plate brimming with greens—a spring salad mix: majestic purple radicchio, forest-green arugula, and ivory endive spears, all lightly dressed with flavorful olive oil and a spritz of lemon juice. (Or perhaps even go European and eat your salad after your main course.) Add a side of fire-roasted red peppers, also bathed in olive oil, and you're off to an incredibly healthy eating journey, in living color. The main course—a hefty plate of homemade pasta (whole wheat, of course), perhaps garnished with clams and bathed in a deep red tomato sauce, topped with leaves of basil and slivers of garlic. Pair the meal with a glass of burgundy-hued red wine and that's *amore*—and that's how you eat for life.

The Prevent a Second Heart Attack plan is largely a vegetarian diet that encourages you to eat more vegetables. Just adding greens and a few additional vegetables to your plate each day can provide your arteries with a steady stream of free-radical-neutralizing, anti-inflammatory agents—plant compounds that will elevate your TAC and give you maximum protection against oxidative stress, the driving force behind atherosclerosis.

I urge you to tap into the plant kingdom's kaleidoscope of colors. Eat your *verdure* and at least five additional deeply colored vegetables every day and you will be taking Mediterranean medicine—a cocktail of phytonutrients that together create a unique protective effect that will support you in your quest to reverse heart disease and greatly reduce your chances of having a second heart attack.

Heart-Healthy Food Number 3: Figs and Other Fruit

Live each season as it passes; breathe the air, drink the drink, taste the fruit, and resign yourself to the influences of each.

—Henry David Thoreau, American author, historian, and poet (1817–1862)

 Eat three fresh fruits (including one traditional Mediterranean fruit— such as a fig) every day.

Companion foods Rx: one vitamin C fruit daily, bringing your total fruit intake to at least three

Primary disease-fighting bioactive compounds:

- Polyphenol antioxidant flavonoids: flavonols (quercetin), anthocyanins (malvidin), flavan-3-ols (epicatechin), flavanones (naringenin)
- vitamins (especially vitamins C and E) and minerals (potassium)
- carotenoids: lycopene, lutein, beta-carotene
- soluble and insoluble fiber

Why do figs garner a place on the Prevent a Second Heart Attack plan food list? Figs, like many of the fruits that Mother Nature has so generously provided us, are nutrient dense, meaning you get a big nutritional bang for your calorie buck. Fruit contains a good amount of fiber, vitamins, and potassium, plus an extraordinary array of potent plaque-fighting polyphenols. These sweet treats should be part of everyone's heart-disease-fighting arsenal. In fact, fruit, and especially dried fruits such as figs—which are denser in antioxidants and fiber than fresh fruit—have a significantly higher quantity of polyphenols than even vegetables.[1] And like all fruit, figs are cholesterol, fat, and salt free. Unfortunately, most Americans are not reaping the benefits of fruit's bounty. Only about 17 percent of us get in the government-recommended daily amount of fruit—at least three servings—with the average American eating less than one serving of fruit per day.[2]

FABULOUS FIGS AND OTHER FRUIT FOR YOUR HEART

Figs, which grow on trees *(Ficus carica),* are one of the first fruits cultivated by human beings and are a staple of the Mediterranean region. Sweet and delicious raw, dried, or as jam, figs are one of the plant kingdom's brightest stars in terms of calcium and fiber content. However, what really labels figs as a bona fide heart attack prevention superfood is their extraordinary amount of carotenoids, most notably lycopene, lutein, and beta-carotene. Few foods on earth are known to contain such an array of heart-health-promoting antioxidants.[3] Dried figs have been scientifically proven to exhibit the highest antioxidant capacity of most commonly eaten dried fruits. Yet despite the fact that dried fruit, and especially figs, is a wonder food for the heart, dried fruit accounts for less than 1 percent of total fruit consumed in the American diet.[4]

Figs must be allowed to ripen fully before being harvested. The purple-skinned, pear-shaped fruits are extremely delicate and too perishable for most markets to keep in stock. That's why 90 percent of all figs are dried upon harvest. So the dried version is what you will most likely be eating. That's not to say you shouldn't eat fresh figs—eat them whenever you can find them (albeit the fresh ones can be rather pricey). Plump, sweet, and filled with hundreds of tiny crunchy seeds, fresh figs are simply a delight.

Fruit for dessert: A habit that reduces heart attack risk

One of the most common components of the Mediterranean eating pattern described in the scientific literature is "fresh fruit for dessert." Adopting this habit will truly help you eat for life—the Mediterranean way. Eat more fruit and you dramatically cut your risk of a heart attack, according to one study out of Spain.[5] Spaniards typically have a very high intake of fresh fruit and fiber, and eating fruit almost exclusively for dessert after the main meal is a traditional Spanish custom.

The Spanish study was a hospital-based "case-control" design, meaning the researchers looked at the eating habits of 171 men and women hospitalized for a recent heart attack (the "cases") and compared them to 171 age-matched men and women (the "controls") who had been admitted to the hospital for noncardiac reasons, such as osteoarthritis or an injury. The findings? Subjects with the highest fruit intake were *86 percent less likely to have had a heart attack* when compared to their low-fruit-eating counterparts.

Fruit's Flavonoid Finesse

Something in that fresh fruit is responsible for keeping our arteries clean. A recent meta-analysis (a compilation of results from several studies totaling 105,000 individuals) found that people who had the highest dietary intake of flavonoids (derived from just a few types of food—fruits, vegetables, tea, and red wine) had a strikingly reduced risk of heart disease.[6] Recall that flavonoids are a subclass of polyphenols, those plentiful and super-heart-healthy plant chemicals found in fruits and vegetables (Figure 7.1). In fact, they are the largest and most diverse subgroup, with more than five thousand disease-fighting phytochemicals identified.[7]

There are six subclasses of flavonoids. The most ubiquitous flavonoids in foods are the flavonols, with quercetin and kaempferol the most abundant flavonols in the diet. The fruits with the greatest amount of quercetin and kaempferol include blueberries, black currants, apples, dark grapes, and apricots. Berries provide the highest level of polyphenols per serving among fruit, yet most Americans don't eat nearly enough.[8] And don't even think about peeling off the skin of that grape or apple—the skin is the most potent source of nutrients. Why? The biosynthesis of the flavonols is stimulated by light, so the flavonols tend to accumulate in the outer tissue.[9] Peel the fruit and you toss out the bulk of the fruit's antioxidant content.

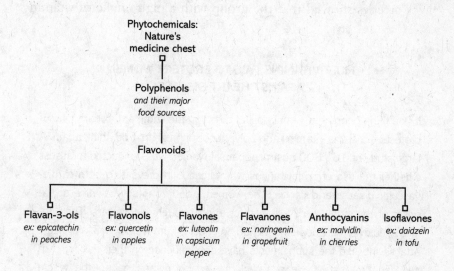

Figure 7.1. Flavonols are the most abundant type of antioxidant flavonoid polyphenols in food. They play a powerful role in the fight against heart disease, with quercetin and kaempferol as the major flavonols in the diet.

Scientific evidence proves that people who eat the most flavonoids are least likely to succumb to a deadly heart attack. The Zutphen elderly study out of the Netherlands, which investigated the eating habits of 805 men age sixty-five to eighty-four, proved this. After five years, researchers found that men who had the highest consumption of flavonoids (quercetin in particular) were *68 percent less likely to die* from heart disease compared to those eating the least amount of flavonoids.[10]

Vitamin C–rich fruits boost heart health

It's not just the flavonoids that have a positive effect on your arteries. A recent study from Ulleval University in Norway reports that eating fruits high in vitamin C such as berries can protect against the progression of atherosclerosis.[11] Four hundred eighty-seven men, with an average age of seventy, completed the three-year study. At the conclusion of the study, an ultrasound of participants' neck arteries showed that the group with a high intake of vitamin

---

MULTIVITAMINS FAIL TO PROTECT WOMEN AGAINST HEART DISEASE

If you think popping a vitamin pill affords you the same antioxidant cardioprotection that the vitamins and polyphenols in fresh fruit do, think again. A large study of 161,808 postmenopausal women was conducted to assess whether the use of multivitamins was effective in preventing both cardiovascular disease and cancer. The women, age fifty to seventy-nine at the onset of the study, were followed for approximately eight years. The findings? Multivitamin supplements had no effect on the women's risk for heart attacks (nor did the supplements have any influence on their risk for cancer). The message? Heart attack prevention means eating the whole fruit—don't waste your money on expensive supplements or deny yourself the pleasure of eating the real thing!

Source: Marian L. Neuhouser et al., "Multivitamin use and risk of cancer and cardiovascular disease in the Women's Health Initiative cohorts,"*Archives of Internal Medicine* 169, no. 3 (2009): 294–304.

C–rich fruit exhibited much less progression of atherosclerotic plaque compared to the other groups.

Conversely, a consistently low level of vitamin C in the bloodstream was shown to almost triple the risk of a heart attack, according to researchers from Finland.[12] More than 1,600 middle-aged men without heart disease living in eastern Finland were followed for eight years. The men with the lowest blood levels of vitamin C had *2.5 times the risk of having a heart attack* compared to men with a higher vitamin C level. But don't use this finding as an excuse to take shortcuts: In this study, taking vitamin C supplements did not have any effect on risk for a heart attack. Nothing compares to whole, fresh fruit, so eat up!

To help you fill your Prevent a Second Heart Attack fruit prescription, consult the following chart to make sure you get in at least one Mediterranean-style fruit and two companion fruits daily.

Mix 'n' Match Your Fruit for Health

Fruit	Daily Serving	Sample Fruits	Primary Disease-Fighting Components
Traditional Mediterranean-style fruit	At least one	Figs, red grapes, olives, pomegranates, mandarin oranges (a variety of clementine), persimmons, cactus pears, loquats, apricots, citrus	Carotenoids *(beta-carotene, beta-cryptoxanthin, lycopene);* flavonoids *(quercetin, kaempferol, myricetin, catechins);* soluble and insoluble fiber
Vitamin C–rich fruits	At least one	Cantaloupe, grapefruit, guavas, kiwi fruit, kumquats, lemons, lychee nuts, oranges, mangoes, peaches, papayas, pineapple, strawberries, tangerines	Vitamin C; flavonoids *(naringenin, quercetin, kaempferol, myricetin);* potassium; soluble and insoluble fiber
Other fruits	At least one	Apples, bananas, berries, cherries, dates, nectarines, plums, prunes, raisins, peaches, pears, starfruit	Soluble fiber *(pectin)* and insoluble fiber; flavonoids *(quercetin, anthocyanins, kaempferol);* vitamin C; potassium

DAILY HEART DISEASE REVERSAL STRATEGY: FRUIT'S CONTRIBUTION

Strategy 1. Boost total antioxidant capacity

Consuming your daily fig and other fruits will supply your body with an extraordinary array of antioxidants including flavonoids, carotenoids, and vitamin C, making a major contribution to your TAC and warding off oxidative destruction. Scientists have investigated what happens in your arteries when you eat a piece of fruit. To explore the blood antioxidant capacity of consuming figs in particular, researchers at the University of Scranton in Pennsylvania administered a glass of soda with or without a serving of dried figs to ten healthy, fasting volunteers. (The carbonated soft drink was used to promote oxidative stress in the arteries.) Blood was analyzed for the antioxidant level at varying intervals for six hours following food consumption. The soda-and-fig-eating group demonstrated a phenomenal 9 percent rise in blood antioxidant level, compared to a drop observed in the soda-only group.[13] Figs contain such powerful antioxidants that they produce a much greater increase in blood antioxidant capacity than even that well-known liquid antioxidant powerhouse, green tea.

Antioxidants in figs protect LDL from free radical attack. The fig group in the University of Scranton study also had a significant enrichment of their LDL cholesterol with antioxidants, which proved to markedly inhibit LDL oxidation (via scavenging of free radicals). This compared to LDL exhibiting severe oxidative damage in the soda group. Oxidative damage modifies LDL cholesterol, and only modified LDL can be engulfed by macrophages in the arterial wall, creating foam cells—the hallmark of atherosclerosis and plaque formation.

Antioxidant vitamins get boost from flavonoids. Flavonoids in figs and other fruits partner with vitamin antioxidants, protecting and extending their usefulness to the body.[14] Vitamin C, for example, is the body's main water-soluble antioxidant in the blood, yet because it is a fast-acting antioxidant, it gets used up fairly quickly. Flavonoids keep the blood level of vitamin C up longer. Thus, to extend the life of vitamin C to fight off free radical attack, it is important to include flavonoids in your daily heart disease antioxidant defense system. Flavonoids also interact with vitamin E, the powerful fat-soluble antioxidant vitamin that helps protect LDL from marauding free radicals. Flavonoids guard against the destruction of vitamin E within the LDL wall and help regenerate the vitamin E once it is used up in LDL's fight against oxidation.[15]

Polyphenols have their maximum concentration in the bloodstream one to two hours after eating and are cleared from the blood within two to four hours of consumption.[16] So don't forget to constantly replenish your arterial antioxidant supply by eating small amounts of polyphenol-rich fruits and vegetables as snacks and in main meals. This will provide your heart with a steady supply of antioxidants to combat oxidative stress throughout the day.

Strategy 2. Protect against endothelial dysfunction

Recall from Chapter 2 that a key early event in the process of atherosclerosis is when an abnormality in the functioning of the inner layer of the artery wall—the endothelium—arises, called *endothelial dysfunction*. Consuming flavonoid-packed fruit can make a dysfunctional endothelium more functional. Quercetin, the main flavonoid polyphenol found in high amounts in plant foods such as apples and onions, has been proven to be a potent anti-inflammatory and antioxidant substance that targets the endothelium—nipping plaque formation right in the bud.[17] What's more, many animal studies have shown that quercetin is a potent coronary *vasodilator*, meaning it has a unique ability to relax the arteries,[18] a beneficial effect for you because stiff arteries are conducive to forming diseased arteries.

A healthy endothelial function is reflected by the inner lining of the artery's ability to loosen up and dilate in response to the increased stress of blood flow, so relaxing your blood vessels is important in your fight against atherosclerosis.

Strategy 3. Lower blood pressure

Consuming your daily fruit prescription will lower elevated blood pressure—a tremendous health concern for cardiac patients, as uncontrolled blood pressure accelerates plaque formation. Let's not forget our key formula from Chapter 1: Reduce systolic blood pressure—the top number—to a normal level (120 mm Hg or less) *and* get LDL cholesterol way down to 70 mg/dL or less.[19]

The popular Dietary Approaches to Stop Hypertension (DASH) diet, which is low in salt and high in fruits and vegetables (nine servings per day), has been proven to reduce high blood pressure without medication.[20] The three key blood-pressure-lowering minerals in the DASH diet are potassium, magnesium, and calcium. The mineral potassium plays an exceptionally large role in lowering blood pressure, and fruits and vegetables are the main food sources of this super-heart-healthy mineral. In the DASH diet, the intake of potassium was 4,700 milligrams per day, which is three times that of the average American diet. Fruits—especially bananas, oranges, and prunes—are loaded with potassium. One banana has almost 500 milligrams. (Of course, greens and other vegetables are also potassium superstars; 1 cup of cooked spinach contains a whopping 839 milligrams, one baked potato 900 milligrams.)

Potassium-to-sodium ratio affects blood pressure. It's well known that excess sodium in the diet is a major cause of high blood pressure, which takes a great toll on your coronary arteries and in turn significantly increases your risk of another heart attack. A new study published in the prestigious *Archives of Internal Medicine* has shown that consuming twice as much potassium as sodium halved subjects' risk of death from heart disease compared to those who ate the most sodium and the least potassium (four times as much sodium as potassium).[21] Keep in mind that most Americans consume far more than the recommended daily limit of 1,500 milligrams of sodium. (A typical restaurant meal may contain more than 4,000 milligrams of sodium—the amount we should consume over *three days*.)

How do you accomplish changing the ratio of potassium to sodium? Simple . . . take a two-step approach: Fill your day with potassium-rich fruits and vegetables and eat as little salt as possible. The best way to reduce your salt intake is to eat fresh, unprocessed foods whenever possible (whole grains, nuts, fruit, vegetables, olive oil). If you eat out, order simple unadulterated foods (salad bar, steamed veggies, grilled fish—plain) and use alternative seasonings to flavor your food (lemon juice, herbs, spices, and vinegars).

Strategy 4. Lose weight

Eating your daily fruit prescription will also help you control your weight, and being overweight is another major risk factor that ups your odds of another heart attack. A recent study found that each daily 100-gram increase in fruit or vegetable intake—approximately one piece of fruit or roughly 1 cup of raw veggies—was associated with a body weight reduction of 500 grams for vegetables and 300 grams for fruit. That equates to a weight loss of a little more than a pound and a half after six months.[22] This may seem like a paltry amount of weight loss, but think again—eating just one piece of fruit and one serving of vegetables a day translates into three pounds a year and thirty pounds a decade. Fiber-rich, low-calorie fruits and vegetables increase feelings of satiety, which helps with weight control. So as you fill up on those low-calorie, antioxidant-packed fruits and veggies, you'll also watch your waistline go down—slowly but surely.

TIPS FOR GETTING IN YOUR DAILY DOSE OF FRUIT

• Make fresh fruit and whole grains standard breakfast fare. Add seasonal berries or dried fruit such as cranberries to your oatmeal (the heart-healthiest breakfast cereal). If you typically drink orange juice at breakfast, switch to eating a whole fruit—this way you get more fiber and flavonoids in fewer calories—a bargain that both your heart and your waistline can appreciate!

• Try fruit for dessert. If you just can't go to bed without a little something sweet, why not try some dried figs? And no, I'm not talking about a certain famous fig cookie, two of which give you a mere 1 gram of fiber (not to mention lots of added sugar, salt, and even some artery-clogging trans fat). Compare that to the real thing—what Mother Nature intended for us to eat—two dried figs, which offer a whopping 5 grams of fiber, a huge cache of blood-pressure-lowering potassium (348 milligrams), and a nice dose of bone-building calcium, with zero added sugar or fat. If it was good enough for Cleopatra, why not give it a try?

• Substitute fruit for fat in baking recipes. Mashed bananas or prune purée works astonishingly well in baked goods. They add moistness with fiber and flavonoids—but without the fat. If you're not a baker, dried figs are a tasty addition to soups or legume dishes and add a hint of sweetness.

• Add figs or other dried fruits like cranberries, apricots, or currants to your dark green leafy salad—a delicious, sweet addition to spruce up the salad as well as give you a feast of antioxidants, especially if you dress the salad with lemon juice and an olive oil vinaigrette.

• Try fruit for snacks, as fresh fruit is ideal when you're on the go. There's nothing like a flavorful, juicy apple to take the edge off your appetite and satisfy a sweet tooth, plus it will give you almost 5 grams of fiber (and included in the fiber, a nice dose of that special brand of LDL-cholesterol-lowering soluble fiber, pectin)—and all this for a measly 80 calories.

• Make fruit easily accessible. Place an eye-appealing bowl of assorted fruit smack dab in the center of high-traffic areas in your house and be sure to grab a piece when you walk by.

• Flavor everything with vitamin C–packed citrus juice: fresh lemon, lime, or orange. For instance, carry a large container of cold water to sip on throughout the day, flavored with fresh lemon or lime juice and a touch of sweetener.

• Buy seasonal fresh fruit—it's refreshing, satisfying, and cost effective, especially in the summer months. Go for the colorful antioxidant-packed berries such as raspberries, blackberries, boysenberries, strawberries, and blueberries. Cherries, peaches, watermelon, cantaloupe, and exotic fruits such as papaya, passion fruit, and mango offer you fiber, vitamin C, and potassium, and all for a low-calorie bargain.

SOMEWHERE OVER THE RAINBOW YOUR DREAMS REALLY WILL COME TRUE

I grew up spending summers on the Jersey shore. I have memories of biting into the deep purple skin of a perfectly ripe plum, having to bend over when eating it so that the incredibly sweet, juicy pulp that poured down my face wouldn't stain my clothes. Ripe, sweet, fragrant, and deliciously healthy, now that's eating well. Red, orange, yellow, purple, and blue . . . find a good purveyor and take the time to choose fresh, seasonal, bright, and attractive fruit in a rainbow of colors and you will reap the phenomenal heart health benefits associated with daily consumption of flavonoid-packed fruit. Remember, when it comes to eating fruits and vegetables and reversing heart disease, more is better—so don't be shy! Nine servings a day may sound like a lot, but scientifically speaking, that's how much you should eat to minimize your risk of disease.[23] Go to the farmer's market, the fruit aisle—anywhere that has fresh, delicious fruit—and stock up! Your heart will thank you.

8

Heart-Healthy Food Number 4: Lentils and Other Legumes

You, who dare insult lentil soup, sweetest of delicacies.

—Aristophanes, Greek playwright (c. 448–380 B.C.)

 Eat lentils or another type of legume every day.

Companion foods Rx: beans and peas (including split peas; broad, navy, great northern, pinto, kidney, red, butter, and black beans; and chickpeas, soybeans, and peanuts)

Primary disease-fighting bioactive compounds:

- Plant protein
- Polyphenol antioxidants: flavonoids (quercetin, anthocyanins)
- Isoflavones (genistein and daidzein), phenolic acids (ferulic acid), and lignans
- Soluble and insoluble fiber

Since the dawn of civilization, legumes have sustained humankind. Legumes are seeds of the Leguminosae family—plants that house their seeds in a double-seamed pod—and include beans, peas, lentils, lupins, soybeans, and peanuts. Lentils are an ultra-lean and remarkably heart-healthy legume—a source of plant protein—providing the backbone for Prevent a Second Heart Attack's primarily plant-based diet. So let's take a closer look at this star of the legume family, the lentil, a spectacularly nutritious (and dirt cheap) plant food extravaganza.

LENTILS: THE LONGEVITY LEGUME

Lentils have been part of the culinary culture of the Mediterranean throughout the ages and are one of the oldest crops cultivated and domesticated by humans. (Lentils, chickpeas, beans, and peas are the most commonly consumed legumes in the Mediterranean basin.[1]) The cultivation of lentils has been traced back as far as 6000 B.C. in parts of the present-day Middle East.[2] Legumes have a colorful history, with four of the most distinguished Roman families named after these seeds: Lentulus (lentil), Fabius (fava bean), Cicero (chickpea), and Piso (pea). The word *lentil* is derived from the Latin word *lens,* as indeed the shape of this bean cousin resembles a biconvex optical sphere, or lens.

These seeds may be petite, but they are nutrition *giants,* loaded with the heart-healthiest of ingredients including fiber, antioxidants, plant protein, vitamins, minerals, and iron—and all this for just pennies on the dollar. What's more, eating legumes such as lentils might just be the dietary secret to longevity.

Australian researchers scientifically confirmed lentils' life-lengthening powers in their study of elderly Greeks. Five groups of subjects (age seventy and older) were drawn from four countries: Greeks in Australia and Greece, Japanese in Japan, Swedes in Sweden, and Anglo-Celtic in Australia. The scientists compared the groups' intakes of various food categories such as vegetables, legumes, dairy, and meat to determine protective dietary predictors among long-lived elderly people of several nations. The single most protective dietary predictor of survival among the elderly, regardless of ethnicity, was found to be simply an abundance of different types of legumes. For every 20-gram increase in daily legume intake, there was an 8 percent reduction in risk of death. No other food group was so strongly predictive of survival into older age, rendering legumes the most important dietary factor in the subjects' longevity. The kind of legume consumed differed among cultures, suggesting that it's not just lentils that confer health benefits. For example, the long-lived Greeks ate lots of lentils, chickpeas, and white beans; the Japanese, an abundance of soy, tofu, natto, and miso; and the Swedes, copious amounts of brown beans and peas.[3]

LEGUMES SLASH HEART DISEASE DEATH RATES

Research published in the prestigious medical journal *Archives of Internal Medicine* supports the spectacular heart health benefits of bulking up the diet with legumes. In a study of 9,632 healthy men and women, followed for a period of nineteen years, individuals consuming legumes four times or more per week compared with less than once a week had a 22 percent lower risk of a cardiac event. The type of legumes participants consumed included dry beans and peas like pinto beans, red beans, black-eyed peas, peanuts and peanut butter. At lunchtime, break out the peanut butter (sans hydrogenated fat) and make a PB & banana sandwich (on whole-grain bread, of course) and you are on the nutritious path to regaining heart health.

Source: Lydia A. Bazzano et al., "Legume consumption and risk of coronary heart disease in U.S. men and women, NHANES I Epidemiologic Follow-Up Study," *Archives of Internal Medicine* 161 (2001): 2573–2578.

LEGUMES' PLANT PROTEIN POWER

Lentils and other legumes are nutritional powerhouses loaded with plant protein—which brings us to the real "meat" of this chapter, the topic of protein. Legumes are Mother Nature's healthy version of meat—you get a nice dose of plant protein but without any of the artery-clogging excess baggage that goes along with animal protein (saturated fat and cholesterol). Plus, you get fiber, vitamins, minerals, and strong antioxidants as a bonus. Americans eat too much animal protein, which tends to be at the center of our plate at breakfast, lunch, and dinner.

The Prevent a Second Heart Attack plan is designed around a "plant-fish" protein philosophy. Choosing the right amount and the right source of protein will make a difference in helping you live better and longer.

Why we need protein

The word *protein* is derived from the Greek word *proteios*, meaning "primary" or "first." Protein is the one nutrient the body requires daily. Why? Because protein is the only nutrient that contains amino acids, which are used to shape protein structures found throughout the body—in skin, hair, nails, muscles, and even the hemoglobin that carries oxygen within red blood cells. Every cell in the body contains protein.

Proteins are made up of chains, and each link in the chain contains one of the twenty types of amino acids. When these links are joined together, the particular combination, sequence, and number of amino acids in each chain distinguishes one type of protein from another. A protein can contain anywhere from two to hundreds to thousands of

---

LENTILS: A HEALTHIER PROTEIN CHOICE THAN STEAK

A cup of lentils served over ½ cup of brown rice contains the same high-quality protein but lacks the fat, cholesterol and calorie overload found in a 9-ounce porterhouse steak.

Lentils and rice	Porterhouse steak
21 grams protein	57 grams protein
2 grams fat	69 grams fat
0 grams saturated fat	27 grams saturated fat
0 milligrams cholesterol	195 milligrams cholesterol
340 calories	870 calories
18 grams fiber	0 grams fiber

The difference is that the steak has its amino acids bundled up with a truckload of artery-clogging saturated fat and cholesterol and has almost three times as many calories! Additionally, the lentils cost about 60 cents a pound compared to $12.99 per pound for the steak. Clearly, the plant protein is healthier for both your heart and your bank account.

amino acids strung together in varying sequences and combinations.

When we eat protein, we are, in effect, digesting or breaking
apart the protein into amino acids. These amino acids enter the
bloodstream to be used as the links for making strands of new proteins. Thus, each kind of protein our cells create is a unique sequence of amino acid placement directed by the blueprint found in
the genes of the cells' DNA.

ALL PROTEINS ARE NOT THE SAME

Complete versus incomplete protein

The human body is capable of making only twelve of the twenty
amino acids required to build new protein structures from scratch.
This means that for good health we must *consume* enough of the
eight essential amino acids that we cannot synthesize on our own.
For these amino acids, it is *essential* we consume them through
diet. On a cellular level, all plant and animal protein contains each
of the twenty amino acids. However, if a certain plant or animal
protein has enough of all the *essential* amino acids—that is to say,
the ones we humans can't make ourselves—then that protein is
considered higher quality or more complete.

Animal proteins are considered high quality because they contain all of the essential amino acids in the right amounts required
by cells to build new protein, which is what makes them *complete*.
Some plant proteins don't have quite enough of one or more essential amino acids for our cells, so we call them *incomplete*. However, plant proteins can be *complementary*, meaning that an
essential amino acid in short supply in one plant protein can be
complemented by finding enough of that amino acid in a *different*
plant protein. A great example of this would be eating legumes and
grains together. Most legumes are deficient in the essential amino
acids methionine and tryptophan. But if you eat those legumes
with a grain, which is rich in methionine and tryptophan, then

you'll be supplied with all the amino acids needed for good health. This is how entire populations have thrived on perfectly complete plant protein combinations such as beans and rice. Nutritionists used to think that complementary plant proteins had to be eaten at the same meal, but this concept is now proven to be invalid. *Our cells get all the essential amino acids required for protein synthesis as long as an array of complementary plant proteins are eaten throughout the day.*

The wisdom of favoring mostly vegetable protein over animal protein

The Prevent a Second Heart Attack plan recommends obtaining most of your daily protein from vegetable sources, with the addition of several weekly servings of animal protein in the form of fish and other seafood (while simultaneously eliminating most other sources of animal protein from your diet such as red meat— beef, pork, veal, lamb, and mutton—and eating skinless white-meat poultry only occasionally). This strategy, concentrating on eating mostly vegetable protein highlighted with several weekly servings of marine protein, forces you to become a more adventurous (and heart-healthier) eater. This is because a diet with too much animal protein (the typical Western diet) contains elements that harm the arteries. Whereas narrowing your protein sources to mostly vegetables, spiced up with the occasional marine source, is an ideal tactic for propelling the reversal of your disease process because both of these types of proteins contain ingredients that participate in your daily heart disease defense system, whereas other protein sources do not.

Excess animal protein is stressful to the body. Of the three macronutrients—carbohydrates, fat, and protein—protein requires the most amount of metabolic work to digest and assimilate. The average diet high in animal protein is chemically different from a plant-based diet in that it generates a large amount of acid. This acidic environment has a detrimental effect on bone density and strength, as the body, in an attempt to neutralize or buffer this excess acid load, compensates by pulling calcium out of the bone. People who routinely consume a high-animal-protein diet have an increased loss of calcium through their urine and a significant amount of bone loss over time, predisposing them to osteoporosis.[4] A plant-based diet has the opposite effect. Eating in this manner supplies the body with a bicarbonate-rich, potassium-rich combination that counteracts acidity and protects and preserves bone mass, promoting long-term skeletal health.[5] Furthermore, potassium, as you learned in Chapter 7, plays a large role in keeping your blood pressure under control.

SOY PRESERVES HEART FUNCTION IN RATS AFTER HEART ATTACK

The soybean is a unique legume. Soybeans can rival any animal protein because they supply all the essential amino acids and in the exact proportion needed by the body. Even better, soy has the added power of antioxidants, cholesterol-lowering fiber, and other plant chemicals that protect against your disease. What's more, eating soy can benefit your injured heart muscle. Brazilian researchers investigated the effect of adding soy protein to the diet of rats in whom a heart attack had been induced. Compared to the rats fed casein (milk protein), the soy-fed rats exhibited improved functioning of the heart ventricle as well as a reduction in oxidative stress. The casein-fed rats, however, showed deterioration of ventricular function.

Source: Martine Kienzle Hagen et al., "Diet with isolated soy protein reduces oxidative stress and preserves ventricular function in rats with myocardial infarction," *Nutrition, Metabolism & Cardiovascular Disease* 19 (2009): 91–97.

There is also a link between animal protein and the formation of kidney stones.[6] Both uric acid and calcium oxalate formation—the building blocks of kidney stones—are increased with a diet high in animal protein. Furthermore, elevated uric acid is the underlying cause of gout, the extremely painful joint inflammatory condition common in overweight men. It has also been suggested, but not conclusively proven, that high-animal-protein diets place an extraordinary amount of stress on and overwork the kidneys over time. What *is* known is that anyone with established kidney disease needs to follow a low-protein diet to prevent further progression of the disease.[7]

DAILY HEART DISEASE REVERSAL STRATEGY: LEGUMES' CONTRIBUTION

Strategy 1. Raise total antioxidant capacity

A daily serving of legumes will make a major contribution to your body's total antioxidant capacity (TAC). Legumes are packed with polyphenol antioxidants: flavonoids (quercetin, anthocyanins); phenolic acids (ferulic acid, vanillic acid); isoflavones (genistein and daidzein); and lignans. (Note that isoflavones and lignans are found primarily in soybeans.) See Figure 10.1.

Beans in particular contain an exceptional amount of antioxidants. There are many varieties of beans, and they come in a mosaic

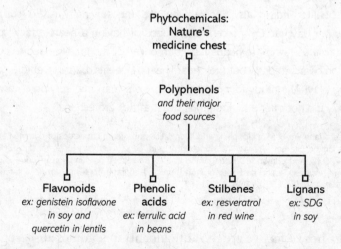

Figure 8.1. Powerful antioxidants are found in legumes. Isoflavones and lignans are two types of polyphenol antioxidants highly concentrated in soybeans.

of deeply hued colors such as the brown and pink mottling characteristic of the pinto bean, the dark red of the kidney bean, the maroon adzuki bean, and the midnight black of the ubiquitous black bean. All of these bean skins contain a large concentration of the colored pigments or powerful antioxidant flavonoids that are superb heart-disease-fighting compounds.

BEANS: A SERVING A DAY KEEPS HEART ATTACKS AT BAY

Beans: peasant food, poor man's meat, *and* the healthy man's staple! Unfortunately, Americans have failed to embrace beans—a tasty, versatile, hearty, and ridiculously inexpensive superfood. Beans contain the most protein of any vegetable; plus, they are loaded with essential B vitamins (especially heart-healthy folate), minerals, and fiber to help you feel full longer. Beans are also a rich source of complex carbohydrates that provide long-lasting energy. The dark varieties of beans such as black beans, pinto beans, and red kidney beans top the U.S. Department of Agriculture's list of foods highest in disease-fighting antioxidants.

Beans also protect against heart attacks, according to a group of researchers at Harvard University who interviewed 2,119 Costa Rican first-heart-attack survivors and compared them to an equal number of matched heart-healthy individuals. People who ate one serving (just ⅓ cup) of beans per day had 38 percent lower odds of having a heart attack compared to those who ate beans less than once per month. No need to overdose on beans to draw out their heart-health benefits, because a little goes a long way! The study found that eating more than one serving of beans per day did not offer any additional heart attack protection.

Sources: Xlanli Wu et al., "Lipophilic and hydrophilic antioxidant capacities of common foods in the United States," *Journal of Agricultural and Food Chemistry* 52, no. 12 (2004): 4026–4037; and Edmond K. Kabagambe et al., "Decreased consumption of dried mature beans is positively associated with urbanization and nonfatal acute myocardial infarction," *Journal of Nutrition* 135 (2005): 1770–1775.

Just how effective are the antioxidants in legumes at scavenging free radicals? Greek scientists decided to investigate this question. Extracts from eleven varieties of Greek legumes (including lentils, white lupin beans, and fava beans) were tested in a lab for antioxidant activity. All the extracts showed significant ability to scavenge free radicals, exerting potent protective activity against DNA damage. Thus, the researchers concluded that legumes' high antioxidant content is one main reason for their heart disease prevention capabilities.[8]

Strategy 2. Control cholesterol and triglycerides

Getting in some legumes every day will lower both your "bad" LDL cholesterol and your triglyceride level. Legumes contain a good deal of soluble fiber, the kind that forms a gel-like substance in the intestinal tract, entrapping cholesterol and ferrying it out of the body. Science supports the notion that eating legumes is effective cholesterol-lowering medication. More than four decades of research has proven that regular consumption of dried legumes, also known as *pulses,* has cardioprotective effects, particularly on the blood cholesterol and triglyceride values. "Dried" beans and peas are actually just the mature forms of legumes and include familiar foods such as kidney beans, black beans, split peas, lentils, and chickpeas. (Fresh green beans, baby lima beans, garden peas, and young soybeans [edamame] are not considered dried beans or pulses but are still foods that have a salutary effect on your arteries.)

Researchers at the University of Kentucky performed a meta-analysis of eleven clinical trials examining the effect of consuming pulses on cholesterol and triglyceride levels. (A meta-analysis is a statistical test that groups the results of multiple studies to come up with one strong conclusion.) The meta-analysis demonstrated that regular intake of pulses lowers LDL cholesterol by an average of 6.2 percent, raises "good" HDL cholesterol by 2.6 percent, and lowers triglycerides by 16.6 percent.[9]

Strategy 3. Lower homocysteine level

Consuming your daily dose of legumes will raise your blood level of an important B vitamin called folate. Folate helps you in your fight against atherosclerosis because it lowers the amount of homocysteine in the blood. Homocysteine is a precarious kind of amino acid that circulates in the bloodstream. A high level of homocysteine has been linked to heart attacks, stroke, and a host of other diseases. Some scientists believe that homocysteine damages the inner lining of the artery and promotes blood clots—two scenarios that increase your risk of a second attack. Your blood level of homocysteine is under your control, because it is greatly influenced by what you eat. Foods high in folic acid can bring a dangerously high homocysteine level down.[10]

Lentils lead the pack in terms of containing more folate than any other plant. The terms *folate* and *folic acid* are often used interchangeably, though they are not the same. *Folate* is the naturally occurring B vitamin found in high concentration in foods such as lentils, chickpeas, and spinach. *Folic acid* refers to the synthetic form of the B vitamin, the kind that is added to foods to fortify them and is also the synthetic form of the vitamin used in formulating supplements.

Strategy 4. Help treat metabolic syndrome and prevent diabetes

Eating your daily legume prescription will lower your fasting insulin level and help manage blood sugar disorders. Legumes are a good source of fiber (both soluble and insoluble), have a low glycemic index, and are rich in complex carbohydrates, all of which prevent blood sugar levels from rising too rapidly after a meal. An elevated fasting insulin level is associated with insulin resistance and metabolic syndrome (a dangerous combination of medical disorders characterized by excess belly fat). Metabolic syndrome is a condition that greatly increases your risk of developing type 2 diabetes, which can severely damage your heart and blood vessels and predispose you to experiencing another cardiac event. How do you know if you have metabolic syndrome? The diagnosis is typically made by your physician if you have three or more of the following conditions:

- Waist greater than 40" for men or 35" for women
- Triglycerides greater than 150 mg/dL or taking medication to lower triglycerides
- HDL cholesterol less than 40 mg/dL for men or 50 mg/dL for women, or taking medications to raise HDL
- Fasting blood glucose over 100 mg/dL, or taking blood-glucose-lowering medication
- Blood pressure of 130/85 or higher, or taking blood-pressure-lowering medication[11]

The simple daily addition of a small amount of legumes such as chickpeas to your day can have a tremendous salutary effect on your blood sugar metabolism. Australian researchers fed forty-five healthy volunteers about 104 grams a day (a little less than ½ cup) of drained, canned chickpeas and analyzed their blood to see the effect. At the end of the twelve-week "chickpea phase," the fasting insulin level of the subjects was significantly reduced compared to the phase in which the subjects followed their usual diet (without chickpeas).[12]

Adding legumes to your diet, especially soybeans and peanuts, can cut your risk of developing type 2 diabetes almost in half, according to a new study by two sets of collaborative researchers from Vanderbilt University and the Shanghai Cancer Institute. The study recruited 64,227 middle-aged healthy Chinese women and followed them for 4.6 years. A high intake of all forms of legumes was associated with a 38 percent decrease in risk, whereas a high intake of soybeans cut the risk of developing type 2 diabetes by 47 percent.[13]

Strategy 5. Improve endothelial function and reduce plaque buildup

Eating soybeans can improve the functioning of the endothelium and reduce the amount of plaque in your arteries. As we all know by now, a poorly functioning endothelium (inner layer of your coronary arteries) is an initiating event in the process of atherosclerosis. Scientists estimate the degree of endothelial dysfunction using a medical test that measures the ability of the vessel to dilate when blood flows through it. The test, typically performed in the main artery of the arm (brachial artery), is called *flow-mediated dilation* (FMD) and is used to evaluate cardiovascular risk. A second test, often performed on the main arteries of the neck, is called *carotid artery intima-media thickness* (C-IMT) and is a surrogate measure of atherosclerosis.

Researchers used these tests to assess the effect of isoflavones on the health of the arteries. Isoflavones, naturally occurring antioxidant polyphenols found in high concentration in soybeans and to a much lesser extent in chickpeas, have highly cardioprotective properties. A study published in the *American Journal of Clinical Nutrition* investigated the effects of soy intake on the arterial blood flow of 126 patients with documented heart disease at high risk for a future cardiac event. The researchers studied their dietary habits for three months. The subjects with the highest isoflavone intake or >13.3 mg/day (one serving of a traditional soy food, such as an 8-ounce glass of soymilk or 4 ounces of tofu, contains approximately 25 milligrams of isoflavones) had a significantly better endothelial function (assessed via better FMD scores) and a reduced amount of neck artery plaque buildup (assessed via lower C-IMT levels) compared to the low-isoflavone eaters.[14]

TIPS FOR GETTING IN YOUR DAILY DOSE OF LEGUMES

• Have a snack of fresh raw veggies dipped in hummus. Hummus is ridiculously easy to make: Simply combine a can of rinsed and drained chickpeas, some tahini, lemon juice, extra virgin olive oil, and garlic in your food processor; whirl away and you're good to go.

• Routinely sprinkle a can of rinsed and drained chickpeas or kidney beans into your salad or daily "greens."

• Eat legume-based soups such as lentil, split pea, black bean, pasta e fagioli ("pasta and beans" in Italian), or minestrone.

• Snack on edamame—delectable baby soybeans often served in the pod—available as an appetizer at Japanese restaurants, or they can be purchased frozen at your local supermarket. (Note that the soybean pods are very fibrous and are not edible.)

• Try meatless vegetarian chili—use two or three different kinds of beans in the recipe instead of the ground beef. Add some shredded soy cheese on top.

• Learn to cook with lentils; they have a rich, nutty flavor and no presoaking is required. Lentils are fast and easy and add flavor to soups, stews, and salads. Spruce up your tomato sauce with lentils and enjoy a fast and delicious heart-healthy meal in minutes.

• Order a three-bean salad at the deli.

• Go vegetarian and opt for a vegetable stir-fry with tofu for dinner.

• Try a handful of soy nuts as a snack.

• Wherever you use cow's milk, replace with light soy milk. And don't forget to use soy milk (instead of water) to cook up your morning bowl of oatmeal.

• Eat a soy- or bean-based veggie burger at your next barbecue and add a side of baked beans.

LUCIFEROUS LEGUMES: LIGHTING YOUR PATH TO WELLNESS

Rustic Italian bean escarole soup, a fava bean appetizer with a smooth Chianti, or perhaps a tasty hummus dip made from ground chickpeas and served with warm olive oil–drenched pita. Legumes—beans, peas, and lentils—are as Mediterranean as apple pie is American. The heart-healthiest traditional Mediterranean style of eating involves fresh and flavorful foods simply prepared. So why get fussy with those American meats, which are so hard to prepare? Instead, why not opt for some vine-ripened tomatoes, onions, and carrots tossed in olive oil, then seasoned with herbs and spices, augmented with lentils, and simmered on the stovetop? Oh, those lovely little lentils . . . for pennies per pound, you get a whole lot of heart-disease-reversing nutrition.

The humble legume is one of the key foods in the Prevent a Second Heart Attack plan. Legumes' complex carbohydrates provide long-lasting energy and plant protein, and unlike animal protein they are rich in plaque-fighting fiber and phytochemicals. Embrace these small life-saving plant proteins and start today to take a giant leap in fighting and even reversing your disease. Now that you have learned about the importance of including plenty of vegetable proteins in your new ultra-heart-healthy eating plan, let's move on to the much heralded (and exquisitely flavorful) primary source of animal protein in the Prevent a Second Heart Attack plan—the pièce de résistance and hallmark of Mediterranean cuisine—fresh and delicious protein from the sea.

Heart-Healthy Food Number 5: Salmon and Other Seafood

Give me a fish and I eat for a day. Teach me to fish and I eat for a lifetime.

—Ancient Chinese proverb

 Eat salmon and other seafood on most days of the week and take one fish oil pill daily.

Companion foods Rₓ: At least three oily fish meals per week and additional seafood as desired:

- Oily fish such as mackerel, halibut, albacore tuna, sardines, or herring
- Additional seafood such as clams, shrimp, octopus, or scallops

Primary disease-fighting bioactive compounds:

- Marine-derived omega-3 fatty acids: eicosapentaenoic acid (EPA) and docosahexaenoic acid (DHA)
- Vitamin D

It's called the "Eskimo factor." As early as 1944, scientists began to document that Greenland Eskimos had virtually no heart disease. This phenomenon occurred despite the fact that the Eskimos ate a diet low in fruits, vegetables, and complex carbohydrates. But they did subsist on a diet loaded with oily seafood such as whale and seal meat—providing the Eskimos with a huge daily dose of fish oil (about 15 grams), rich in the superbly heart-healthy marine omega-3 polyunsaturated fatty acids (PUFAs).[1] Over the past several decades, however, the Greenlanders' lifestyle has become increasingly Westernized, resulting in an increase in risk factors for heart disease and an expected corresponding increase in mortality rate.[2] Sadly, just as with the Tepehuanos Indians discussed in Chapter 1, as soon as the Greenlanders adopted our Westernized eating habits, their health began to suffer.

Omega-3 fish fat can protect against a second heart attack by targeting the three key areas of vulnerability in you, our *trilogy of vulnerability*:

1. *Vulnerable plaque*—omega-3s slow down the disease process and can even promote reversal of atherosclerosis

2. *Vulnerable heart muscle*—omega-3s protect against electrical disturbances of the heart (arrhythmias)

3. *Vulnerable blood*—omega-3s thin the blood, making platelets less likely to stick together and form clots[3]

So for now, let's "go fish" and focus our discussion on the spectacular benefits of eating omega-3-packed fish on most days of the week, along with taking your supplementary prescription fish oil capsule.

> The best sources of omega-3 fatty acids are the species of fish with darker meat, such as salmon, mackerel, lake trout, herring, sardines, and albacore tuna.

FISH: THE WONDER FOOD

Fish and especially the fatty types of fish that swim in the deep, cold waters of the sea are human beings' primary source of the key fatty acids known to enhance human health: the twin polyunsaturated or "long-chain" omega-3 fats eicosapentaenoic acid (EPA) and docosahexaenoic acid (DHA). Remember how we as humans can't synthesize all the essential amino acids that make up proteins? Well, similarly, fish can't synthesize the fatty acids that we've come to associate with them. Instead, they accumulate these omega-3 fatty acids into their own fat cells as predatory species, by eating aquatic microorganisms such as certain types of microalgae and krill—the original producers of the omega-3 fatty acids EPA and DHA. (So if you can't bear the thought of eating fish or popping fish pills, perhaps an algae appetizer?)

Another reason to eat fish, particularly the fatty types like salmon, is that fish provides a rich cache of vitamin D—the hottest nutrition topic at the moment, linked to many positive traits such as cardiovascular health and living a longer life. Experts now consider vitamin D a highly cardioprotective nutrient that protects against atherosclerosis by taming inflammation and blocking plaque proliferation.[4] An explosion of new research links vitamin D deficiency with a propensity to develop coronary artery disease. Vitamin D deficiency is quite prevalent in the United States, which experts believe may be a strong contributing factor to the epidemic of heart disease in this country. A recent study of 1,739 offspring from the Framingham Heart Study's original participants, followed over seven years, proved this point. Researchers found that the risk of cardiovascular events was twice as high in those with vitamin D deficiency (blood levels of vitamin D of less than 15 nanograms per milliliter [ng/mL]) compared to those with higher blood levels of vitamin D (more than 27 ng/mL).[5]

Vitamin D is an unusual nutrient because it is a vitamin but acts more like a hormone. In fact, its name refers to two types of inactive provitamins known as the *D precursors:* D2 (ergocalciferol) and D3 (cholecalciferol), which are converted from the provitamin forms to their active form by the liver and kidneys. We obtain vitamin D from food, but we also manufacture it when our skin cells

---

LOW VITAMIN D BOOSTS HEART DISEASE DEATH RISK

Inadequate dietary intake of vitamin D along with inadequate sun exposure cumulates in vitamin D deficiency. A recent study of 3,400 older Americans found that compared to people with optimal vitamin D status, those with low vitamin D *had a significantly greater risk of dying from heart disease.* Thus, studies are accumulating suggesting that vitamin D status affects cardiovascular health. You should know, however, that the heart health benefits of raising your level of vitamin D remain far from proven. Despite the preliminary nature of the research, at this time it appears prudent for me to encourage you to ask your doctor to perform a blood test to assess your vitamin D status and to boost your level if it is low.

Vitamin D measurements are reported in either nanograms per milliliter (ng/mL) or nanomoles per liter (nmol/L). A measurement of 25-hydroxy vitamin D, or 25-OH D, level with a value of less than 15 ng/mL (37.5 nmol/L) is deemed by the National Institutes of Health as a deficiency. How high should you go? The scientific consensus points to a blood level of vitamin D that is between 35 and 40 ng/mL (90 and 100 nmol/L) for preventive health.

One simple way to potentially build up your arsenal for fighting off that second heart attack is to get in enough of this important vitamin. The Prevent a Second Heart Attack plan's vitamin D–boosting strategy recommends a triple-pronged approach: Eat your fatty fish prescription and take your daily exercise outside so that you get some sunshine every day. It's tough to consume enough vitamin D in the diet, and many of us residing in northern climates do not get enough sunshine during winter months (or we block the vitamin D–building ultraviolet B light with sunscreen), so I suggest you consider taking a daily supplement (under your doctor's supervision) with 1,000–2,000 international units (IU) of vitamin D, just in case. And make sure that the supplement you take is the vitamin D3 form of the vitamin (cholecalciferol) and *not* D2 (ergocalciferol)!

Sources: Adit A. Ginde et al., "Prospective study of serum 25-hydroxyvitamin D level, cardiovascular disease mortality, and all-cause mortality in older U.S. adults," *Journal of the American Geriatric Society* 57 (2009): 1595–1603; and Mark A. Moyad, "Vitamin D: A rapid review," *Urologic Nursing* 28, no. 5 (2008): 343–349, 384.

are exposed to the sun (vitamin D is also called "the sunshine vita-min"). Food sources of vitamin D include fatty fish such as salmon, tuna, and sardines *(fatty fish is the only naturally rich food source of vitamin D),* fortified dairy products, some soy products, and forti-fied ready-to-eat cereals. Certain brands of orange juice are also fortified with vitamin D. If you haven't guessed already, *fortified* means that the vitamin D was added in artificially.

THE SCIENCE BEHIND EATING FISH FOR A HEALTHY HEART

Many population studies reveal that people who eat a diet high in fish are at much lower risk of having or dying from a heart attack, including Harvard's famed Nurses' Health Study. The Nurses' Health Study is an ongoing long-term study following the lifestyle habits and disease rates of more than 84,000 American women nurses between ages thirty-four and fifty-nine, all in good health at the time of recruitment. In one segment of the study, there were 1,513 recorded incidents of either nonfatal heart attacks or deaths from heart disease. Women who consumed fish five or more times per week lowered the risk of a cardiac event by an impressive 34 percent and the risk of dying by 32 percent compared with women who rarely ate fish.[6] Since the late 1980s, thousands of other scien-tific studies have confirmed that omega-3 fat consumed from either eating fish or taking supplements reduces the risk of having another cardiovascular event such as a heart attack, stroke, and even death by almost 50 percent.[7]

We have known for decades about the power of fish to cut the risk of a second heart attack. Remember from Chapter 3 that heart attack survivors in the famous DART study who were advised to eat two to three portions of fatty fish per week *cut their risk of death by 29 percent* during the first two years following their heart attack compared to the heart patients not given the fish-eating advice.[8]

A new, extensive study published in the *Journal of the American College of Cardiology* goes on to say that eating fish can seriously reverse the course of heart disease. The authors found "compelling evidence" from data of almost forty thousand participants that omega-3 fish oil provides maximal cardioprotection in the treatment of those with existing atherosclerosis.[9] What's more, omega-3 fish fats have also been proven to slow the progression of atherosclerosis in individuals with diagnosed coronary artery disease.[10] So, regardless of what you may have heard about eating fish in the past, clearly, it is time to make fish your routine entrée selection.

FISHING FOR A LONGER LIFE

A recent study backs up the notion that eating fish affects longevity and de-clogs arteries. Researchers compared the degree of plaque buildup in the arteries of middle-aged Japanese men with that of middle-aged white American and Japanese American men living in the United States. Scientists found that the Japanese men, who have one of the highest fish intakes in the world, had twice the amount of heart-healthy omega-3 fish fat in their bloodstream compared to the Americans. It was also shown that the Japanese men had a correspondingly low level of atherosclerosis in their arteries. The Japanese American men and white American men both exhibited a similarly high degree of atherosclerosis.

The fact that the Japanese had almost no evidence of disease yet the Japanese Americans had high rates of atherosclerosis indicates that genetics is not a protective factor in disease risk. The researchers concluded that eating fish year in and year out protects against the development of atherosclerosis.

Source: Akira Sekikawa et al., "Marine-derived Ω-3 fatty acids and atherosclerosis in Japanese, Japanese-American, and white men," *Journal of the American College of Cardiology* 52 (2008): 417–424.

Fish fat plus statin dramatically lowers risk of coronary event

The enormous Japanese EPA Lipid Intervention Study began in 1999 and was designed to examine whether administering an omega-3 fish oil supplement (1.8 grams per day of EPA) together with a low-dose statin drug (either Pravachol or Zocor) would have any additive benefit in the secondary prevention of heart disease. The study involved 18,645 participants who were divided into two groups—statin-only group or statin-plus-fish-oil-pill group—and followed for 4.5 years. The results were spectacular, especially among subjects who had a history of coronary artery disease. In that group, people who took both fish oil *and* a statin had a *19 percent reduction of risk* of having another major coronary event (defined as having another fatal or nonfatal heart attack, sudden cardiac death, uncontrolled angina, or bypass surgery) compared to the people who took a statin only.[11]

HOW MUCH OMEGA-3 IS ENOUGH?

The American Heart Association currently endorses the use of omega-3 fish fats (EPA and DHA) for individuals with known coronary artery disease in a dose of approximately 1 gram per day of a mixture of EPA and DHA. They suggest, however, that ideally heart patients should obtain their daily fish omega-3s from the consumption of oily fish (1 gram of EPA/DHA can be obtained from eating about 3.5 ounces of oily fish such as salmon, Atlantic mackerel, or sardines) as opposed to popping the pills. The AHA states that the use of fish oil capsules is also acceptable but should be considered only in consultation with the patient's physician.[12]

Is there danger in eating too much omega-3 fat?

Concerns that excess omega-3 DHA and EPA could interfere with blood clotting, particularly in patients taking blood-thinning medication such as aspirin, Coumadin, or Plavix, prompted the AHA to issue a warning that taking more than 3 grams of omega-3 fish oil a day *in capsules* could cause excessive bleeding in some people. However, a recent report on potential adverse effects of omega-3 fatty acids concluded that there is virtually no increased risk of excessive bleeding in patients taking up to 7 grams per day of fish oil capsules—even when taken in conjunction with other anti-blood-clotting medications.[13] The bottom line is, you shouldn't worry about getting *too* much fish oil—just worry about whether you're getting *enough*.

What if you have high triglycerides?

According to the AHA, a heart patient who has elevated triglycerides should take 2 to 4 grams of EPA and DHA in capsule form, under a physician's care. However, that amount may not be enough to achieve meaningful triglyceride-lowering results, according to a review published in the journal *Mayo Clinic Proceedings*. The authors of *that* study prescribe between 3 and 4 grams daily of EPA and DHA, in capsule form, for patients with high triglyceride levels.[14]

FOOD, SUPPLEMENTS, OR BOTH?

Fish oil supplements are a highly cost-effective means of cutting your risk of a second and fatal heart attack.[15] But is it better to get your omega-3s by popping pills, eating fish, or both? Ideally, it is best to eat salmon, sardines, herring, or other oily fish, along with other seafood, on most days of the week. By choosing fish as your protein source over, say, chicken, you will be getting a double benefit—a good source of protein *and* omega-3 fat. That said, eating that much fish can be difficult on a practical level—I'd hate for you to get sick of sardines! So, just to be safe, you should consult with your cardiologist about taking an adjunct fish oil supplement, in order to get the optimal omega-3 fatty acid target of at least 1 gram of EPA/DHA per day.

Lovaza (GlaxoSmithKline), formerly known as Omacor, is the brand name of the prescription fish oil supplement and is guaranteed by the Food and Drug Administration to be a safe, high-quality fish oil, free of contaminants and impurities, and to contain exactly what is on the label. One Lovaza capsule provides approximately 900 milligrams of mixed EPA and DHA omega-3 fatty acids.

(*Note:* Prescription fish oil supplements are preferable to over-the-counter supplements, which can vary in quality, purity, and dosage.) The *Mayo Clinic Proceedings* review of the use of omega-3 fatty acids stated that individuals with diagnosed coronary artery disease *must* use fish oil supplements if they are to reach the recommended daily dosage of DHA and EPA.[16] The U.S. Food and Drug Administration (FDA) has limited approval of Lovaza for the treatment of adult patients diagnosed with very high (≥ 500 mg/dL) triglyceride levels. Therefore, you need to discuss with your personal physician whether this prescription is right for you.

The bottom line: Getting your weekly fish prescription from food is ideal, because populations that *eat* a diet high in fish have the lowest death rates from heart disease. However, I recommend that you take a daily prescription fish oil pill as an adjunct to your healthy diet—under your doctor's supervision. Just be sure to consume *at least* 1 gram per day of EPA and DHA (the amount in a small piece of salmon) any way you can, because fish oil is your heart's best friend.

DAILY HEART DISEASE REVERSAL STRATEGY: FISH OIL'S CONTRIBUTION

Strategy 1. Decrease progression and stabilize vulnerable plaque

As previously mentioned, consuming your omega-3 fish oil prescription will decelerate atherosclerosis and reduce the likelihood of developing new plaque in your coronary arteries.

How does fish oil affect vulnerable plaque? According to the extraordinary findings from a study out of the United Kingdom, fish oil readily incorporates into advanced plaque, changing the structure of the plaque and stabilizing it. Researchers randomly administered a daily dose of one of three types of oil—fish oil (1.4 grams per day of omega-3 EPA and DHA), sunflower oil, or a soybean/palm oil blend—to 188 patients with diagnosed advanced coronary artery disease, for an average of forty-two days. At the end of the treatment period, a detailed examination of the patients' neck (carotid) arteries showed that of the three types of oil, only the fish oil incorporated itself into the plaque, enhancing its stability. The fish oil plaque clearly differed from the plaque in the other groups. The stabilizing effect included thicker fibrous caps, fewer macrophage scavenger cells within the intima, and a *complete absence of inflammation.*[17] So put out the flames of inflammation smoldering within your coronary arteries by eating and taking your soothing, plaque-stabilizing, fish fat!

Strategy 2. Reduce your risk of sudden death

Eating your fish oil prescription will stabilize a vulnerable heart muscle by decreasing your risk of arrhythmias (irregular heartbeats), thereby preventing *sudden cardiac death.*[18] Sudden cardiac death (SCD), also called *sudden arrest,* is different from a heart attack. A heart attack occurs when heart muscle tissue dies because of lack of oxygenated blood flow. A heart attack can cause SCD, but the two are not synonymous. SCD occurs when the heart abruptly stops functioning or pumping, which is frequently due to a disturbance in the normal electrical rhythm of the heart (electrical chaos). The most common fatal arrhythmia is known as *ventricular fibrillation.*

Ninety percent of people who die of SCD have evidence of plaque in two or more coronary arteries. Thus, the most common underlying cause of SCD is coronary artery disease. In fact, people who have had a previous heart attack where the blockage resulted in death of a small patch of heart muscle and subsequent scarring are at increased risk of SCD.[19] As a heart disease survivor, you should take extra precautions against arrhythmias—because you're at a much higher risk for SCD. Why fish oils have this powerful anti-arrhythmic effect is still a bit of a mystery—but research proves that fish oil works.

Strategy 3. Lower your triglyceride level

As you now know, high triglycerides greatly increase your risk of a second heart attack. They fuel plaque buildup by creating inflammation at the level of the endothelium, increasing the number of adhesion molecules that surface from endothelial cell walls, increasing the production of new foam cells in the arterial intima, and increasing the proportion of small, dense LDL particles (the dangerous kind that are more susceptible to oxidation).[20] How high is too high? The AHA classifies a blood triglyceride level of less than 150 mg/dL as normal. If your triglycerides are too high, consider consulting with your cardiologist about upping your daily prescription fish oil supplement dosage. As discussed previously, AHA guidelines state that patients who need to lower their triglycerides should consume 2–4 grams of EPA/DHA from supplements under a physician's care,[21] but research and many physicians recommend an even higher dosage.

Strategy 4. Reduce inflammation

As you learned in Chapter 2, inflammation plays a critical role in initiation and progression of atherosclerosis as well as in vulnerable plaque rupture. What you may not know is that getting in your daily marine-derived omega-3 fatty acid prescription will provide your arteries with a variety of anti-inflammatory effects such as improved functioning of the endothelium, reduced oxidative stress, and reduced blood clotting.[22]

Omega-3 fish oils affect your cells' production of *eicosanoids*—hormonelike substances that regulate many bodily functions such as the tendency of blood to clot or the arteries to either dilate or constrict. Eicosanoids are formed from one of the two types of essential fatty acids: omega-3 or omega-6 fats. (*Essential* means we must get the nutrient in our diet for good health because our bodies can't make it.) These fats compete with each other metabolically to produce different types of eicosanoids. Therefore, if you eat more omega-3 fat, your cells will make more of the heart-healthy "good" eicosanoids that thin the blood and promote relaxed arteries, whereas if you eat more omega-6 fat (ubiquitous in the American food supply—such as in vegetable oils and many processed foods) and not enough omega-3 fat, your cells will produce the more inflammatory kinds of eicosanoids that promote blood clotting and constriction of the arteries.

Eating omega-3 fish fat will also lessen inflammation at the site of atherosclerosis by soothing your "dysfunctional" endothelium, making it more "functional." Omega-3 fats boost cells' production of nitric oxide—the natural relaxation chemical that also contributes to widened, relaxed arteries—plus it curbs adhesion molecules so that less immune system cells stick to the artery wall. Finally, omega-3 fatty acids have been proven to quench those highly damaging molecules that play such an active role in propagating oxidative stress. (Remember, oxidative stress accelerates plaque progression by promoting oxidation of LDL cholesterol, foam cell formation, and vulnerable plaque instability.[23])

Strategy 5. Thin your blood

Eating marine-derived omega-3 fatty acids will help make your vulnerable blood less vulnerable. The Greenland Eskimo research showed us decades ago that consuming a high amount of omega-3 fish fat works on the blood, specifically the platelets (those small pieces of cells that stick together to form clots that form a "stopper" in your artery). Eskimo blood was very "thin," meaning the platelets didn't stick together well, which contributed to the rarity of heart disease in the Eskimo people at the time of the study.[24]

WHAT ABOUT MERCURY?

One potential danger of eating a high-fish diet is exposure to unacceptable levels of toxic contaminants such as mercury. Mercury is released into the environment from natural as well as industrial sources, including the burning of fossil fuels and solid wastes and the disposal of mercury-containing products such as certain types of thermometers and fluorescent bulbs. Exposure to excess amounts of mercury can damage the nervous system. Nearly all fish contains a small amount of methylmercury (which is just a fancy way of describing mercury that has accumulated in bodies of water). Mercury contamination is a problem only when high levels accumulate in the flesh of fish such as in older, larger types of predator fish like tuna (albacore, bluefin, bigeye, and yellowfin), swordfish, marlin, and shark.

Methylmercury exposure ups your risk of dying from heart disease. New research has shown that increased exposure to methylmercury in men can promote the development of heart disease and increase the risk of death.[25] In the United States, fish safety is regulated by both the Food and Drug Administration (FDA) for commercial and marine fish and the Environmental Protection Agency (EPA) for sport-caught fish. The EPA and FDA have issued an advisory directed specifically toward women who may become pregnant, women who are pregnant, nursing mothers, and young children.[26] The advisory states that this population should not eat shark, swordfish, king mackerel, or tilefish.

A review of fish intake, contaminants, and human health published in the *Journal of the American Medical Association* suggests that individuals who eat high amounts of fish should limit their intake of the species highest in mercury levels.[27] Omega-3-rich fish and seafood *lowest in mercury* include salmon, shrimp, sardines, trout, herring, and oysters. Prescription fish oil supplements contain negligible amounts of mercury.[28] Other steps you can take to lessen exposure to contaminated fish include eating fish caught from a variety of different locales and eating open-ocean, deep-water fish more often than freshwater fish.

The following chart lists the best fish and seafood choices in terms of omega-3 EPA and DHA content (in descending order).

Fishing for Health	
Fish	**EPA/DHA (g/3-oz. portion)**
Mackerel, Atlantic	1.954
Anchovies, canned in oil, drained	1.746
Salmon, Atlantic, farmed	1.671
Salmon, chinook	1.659
Herring, Atlantic	1.336
Salmon, Atlantic, wild	1.221
Sablefish	1.185
Tuna, bluefin	0.998
Salmon, sockeye	0.996
Salmon, coho, wild	0.923
Sardines, Atlantic, canned in oil, drained	0.834
Trout, rainbow, farmed	0.789
Tuna, white, canned in water	0.733
Oysters, Pacific	0.584
Swordfish	0.543
Rainbow trout, wild	0.499
Shrimp	0.408
Lobster	0.317
Catfish, channel, wild	0.310
Halibut	0.308
Catfish, channel, farmed	0.233
Grouper	0.210
Flatfish (flounder and sole)	0.169
Haddock	0.157
Cod, Atlantic	0.156
Octopus	0.134
Clams	0.121

Note: Omega-3 calculations are for raw seafood (except canned).

Source: U.S. Department of Agriculture Nutrient Data Laboratory, http://www.ars.usda.gov/main/site_main.htm?modecode=12-35-45-00.

SIZING UP SALMON: WILD OR FARMED?

Both wild and farmed salmon contain large amounts of the ultra-heart-healthy (and brain-healthy) fats: omega-3 EPA and DHA. There has been concern regarding the high level of toxic environmental pollutants found in some farm-raised salmon, namely mercury and polychlorinated biphenyls (PCBs); however, these concerns are overblown. Both farm-raised and wild salmon contain well below the federal limits of mercury. Regarding PCBs, the high level in farm-raised salmon has been linked to European-raised salmon, whereas the farm-raised salmon from Chile and Canada (the two nations from which the United States receives 90 percent of its salmon) is significantly lower.

Salmon is the most affordable and richest source of omega-3 fatty acids for people living in the United States. Eat wild salmon (fresh or frozen) if you can get it; if not, farmed is perfectly fine. A reliable way to ensure that you are getting wild salmon is to buy canned Alaskan salmon. Eat at least eight ounces of this safe, nutrient-packed protein per week, which guarantees you'll receive approximately 500 milligrams of EPA and DHA per day (farmed Atlantic salmon) or about 300 milligrams of EPA and DHA per day (wild coho or sockeye salmon). *The health risks of not eating fish are far greater than the exaggerated risk of eating farm-raised fish, so go fish for better heart health and eat salmon.*

Source: Charles R. Santerre, "Wild versus farm-raised salmon: Health benefits and risks," *Sports, Cardiovascular, and Wellness Nutritionists (SCAN) PULSE* 27, no. 4 (2008): 1–5.

CHOLESTEROL CONCERNS

You learned in Chapter 4 that dietary cholesterol intake should be kept to a minimum for heart health. Does this mean you should cut shellfish like shrimp and lobster out of your diet? Absolutely not. The fact is, we tend to eat *much smaller portions* of fish and shellfish than other types of animal protein, making their cholesterol counts much less of a concern. If you compare a typical serving of shrimp (3 ounces, 80 calories, 0 grams saturated fat,

166 milligrams cholesterol) with a typical restaurant serving of prime rib (10 ounces, more than 1,000 calories, 40 grams saturated fat, 240 milligrams cholesterol), you'll understand why you can enjoy the fruit of the sea without breaking the cholesterol bank.

Keep in mind that a single egg yolk contains more than 200 milligrams of cholesterol. Eat just one and you are over the government's recommended daily limit for controlling "bad" LDL cholesterol. Aim for keeping your dietary cholesterol intake *below 200 milligrams per day,* a goal that can easily be accomplished the Mediterranean way by occasionally enjoying a small amount of lean fish or shellfish (or, if you don't want to say good-bye to the incredible, edible egg, just go for the whites).

Isn't a vegan diet better for reversing heart disease?

As I'm sure you all know by now, I am *not* an advocate of spartan, super-low-fat, or restrictive diets. They're unnecessary and they work only if you follow them to a T, which most people can't! Many individuals choose veganism as a lifestyle—for either religious or philosophical reasons. You may be considering it for health reasons. A vegan diet consists of 100 percent plant protein (no dairy, eggs, or fish). If followed correctly, a vegan diet will provide you with sufficient amino acids—but only if you eat a varied diet of plant proteins and consume enough calories throughout the day. As far as treating heart disease goes, some of these strict, ultra-low-fat vegetarian plans have scientific data showing reversal of atherosclerotic plaque. However, they are tough diets to adhere to, and often they ban or severely restrict many of the heart-healthy favorites advocated in this book such as red wine, fish, nuts, and olive oil. Most important, though, *the bulk of the scientific research shows that a Mediterranean style of eating combined with physical activity is the better lifestyle plan for preventing a second heart attack.* If you're not a vegan by choice—that is to say, if you're considering it only because the doctor told you to—I say, don't! Incorporate a *sea* of change in your mindset, and your heart and taste buds will thank you for it.

TIPS FOR GETTING IN YOUR WEEKLY DOSE OF FISH

Fish and seafood can be divided into two general categories: fatty omega-3-rich fish and lean, low-calorie whitefish and shellfish. As you know, the fattier, cold-water fish are richest in omega-3 EPA/DHA fat. A variety of these deep-sea oily fish, such as salmon, tuna, halibut, and mackerel, should be consumed at a minimum of three meals per week. Fatty or low fat, *choose both types of fish on most days of the week as your marine protein source,* because all types of fish contain EPA and DHA, although some types (oily fish) house substantially higher quantities. Getting in your fish prescription is easier than you think. Here's how.

• Go to your local fishmonger and be sure to buy really fresh fish, fish that doesn't have a fishy smell. Don't be shy about asking to smell the fish before purchasing. I buy fish that's right off the boat—in bulk—take it home, cut it into individual servings, wrap in wax paper, label, and freeze.

• If you eat out, frequent a steak house, where you can almost always find salmon or a tuna steak on the menu. Just be sure to order it grilled and simply dressed with a squeeze of fresh lemon.

• Consider a can of water-packed albacore tuna served over your greens for lunch with olive oil vinaigrette—instead of a sandwich of cold cuts.

• Contrary to popular belief, both deep-sea cold-water fish and freshwater fish from cold waters (such as lake herring, lake trout, and whitefish) are good sources of healthful omega-3 fatty acids. Buy them fresh or frozen; bake, grill, or broil the fish (instead of deep-frying) for maximum heart health benefits.

DON'T FRY YOUR FISH!

In a study of almost five thousand adults over age sixty-five, researchers at Harvard University found that people who ate fried fish and fish sandwiches (fish burgers) more than once per week had a 44 percent *greater* risk of having an ischemic stroke (caused by atherosclerosis in a blood vessel leading to the brain) than those who rarely ate their fish fried. Participants who ate baked or broiled fish five or more times a week had a 30 percent *reduced risk* of ischemic stroke.

Source: Dariush Mozaffarian et al., "Fish consumption and stroke risk in elderly individuals," *Archives of Internal Medicine* 165 (2005): 200–206.

• Low-fat fish and seafood (whitefish and shellfish) can also be enjoyed at several meals over the course of the week (in addition to your oily fish prescription). Some examples are tilapia, flounder, clams, and shrimp. Next time you eat Italian, order pasta (whole wheat) with a small amount of shellfish—in red sauce—as your entrée.

• Both squid and octopus are common ingredients in Mediterranean cookery. Go to a Greek restaurant and you will find a varied selection of seafood appetizers or meze on the menu. Try my favorite, Htapothi sti Skhara: flame-grilled octopus seasoned with only olive oil and lemon. *Nosthimia!* (Greek for delicious!)

MEND A BROKEN HEART: EAT FISH

If you were to visit Crete, you would most likely sit down at a seaside restaurant to a mouthwatering meal of grilled fish—right off the boat: perhaps a thick, juicy halibut steak (providing you with half your daily fish oil prescription) seasoned with nothing more than a drizzle of olive oil, fresh garlic, a squeeze of lemon juice, and accompanied by the ubiquitous greens. This is the Mediterranean answer to meat. Or perhaps you might savor an exquisitely succulent fish stew, overflowing with the bounty of the sea—clams, fish fillet, and scallops simmered in a garlic, olive oil, and tomato-based stock, a meal that will give you all the protein you need with half the calories and twice the taste of beef.

If you compare the nutrient value of meat and fish, you will find that fish is clearly the superior choice—exceptionally low in artery-clogging saturated fat, yet providing an excellent source of vitamins, minerals, and high-quality protein. Marine protein supplies the full range of essential amino acids, in the right proportions, to support bodily processes—plus it will give you a nice dose of the spectacularly heart-healthy superfat: omega-3 fatty acids.

I urge you to become a "vegaquarian" and mend your broken heart by following the Prevent a Second Heart Attack plant/fish protein philosophy. Eat a small piece of fish on most days of the week and take your daily fish pill and you will be taking advantage of the enormous amount of cardioprotection that the fish omega-3 fatty acids DHA and EPA have to offer.

Heart-Healthy Food Number 6: Walnuts and Flaxseeds

Tell me what you eat, and I will tell you what you are.

—Jean Anthelme Brillat-Savarin, French gastronome and author (1755–1826)

 Eat a handful of walnuts (2.6 grams of ALA) every day.

Companion foods Rx: 1½ tablespoons of ground flaxseeds (2.2 grams of ALA) every day; aim for consuming a total of at least 4 grams of ALA per day

Primary disease-fighting bioactive compounds:

- Plant-derived omega-3 fatty acid: alpha-linolenic acid (ALA)
- Nonflavonoid polyphenol antioxidants—ellagic acid and gallic acid
- Arginine
- Vitamin E

ALA: THE "OTHER" OMEGA-3 STAR

Alpha-linolenic acid, or ALA, is the name of the omega-3 fatty acid derived from plants. Mounting research continues to prove that this cousin of the more-celebrated marine-derived omega-3 fats (EPA and DHA) is also powerful medicine for promoting cardiovascular health. Plant- and marine-derived omega-3 fats work in slightly different ways to fight atherosclerosis. The longer-chain

---

SAVING THE DAY WITH ALA

Studies show that people who eat an ALA-rich diet are less likely to suffer a fatal heart attack. In a subset of the Cardiovascular Health Study, blood was drawn and analyzed from a group of 179 older men and women who had suffered either a fatal or nonfatal heart attack (blood was taken approximately 2 years before their event). The level of omega-3 and omega-6 fats were measured in cells circulating in the subjects' blood and compared to blood samples of 179 age-matched controls. (This type of study is called a *case-control study,* in which researchers look back on subjects who already have a disease to see if they possess characteristics in common that differ from people who don't have the disease.) The results? Researchers found that participants with a high blood level of ALA had a 50 percent decrease in risk of death from a cardiac event. On the other hand, participants with a high blood level of the omega-6 fat linoleic acid (LA) had more than twice the risk of a fatal cardiac event compared to those with lower levels.

ALA intake can also have a powerful impact on lowering your odds of having a second heart attack. Recall from Chapter 3 the Lyon Heart Study, which demonstrated the superb cardioprotective effect of getting in the "other" omega-3 fat, ALA. In a group of 608 heart patients following an ALA-rich Mediterranean diet, a follow-up at twenty-seven months showed a *73 percent reduction* in risk of another heart attack and a 70 percent overall decrease in mortality compared to the group not following the diet. The subjects in the experimental group had attained a low consumption of LA compared to their consumption of omega-3 ALA—a ratio of 4:1—and a total ALA intake recorded as *triple* that of the control group. This illustrates that to get your ratio more in balance, simply cut out most of the foods that contain LA (such as safflower, cottonseed, and other typical salad dressing oils) and get in your daily omega-3 prescription of both EPA/DHA fish oil and plant ALA (at least 4 grams daily).

Sources: Rozenn N. Lemaitre et al., "Polyunsaturated fatty acids, fatty ischemic heart disease, and nonfatal myocardial infarction in older adults: The Cardiovascular Health Study," *American Journal of Nutrition* 77 (2003): 319–325; and Michel de Lorgeril et al., "Mediterranean alpha-linolenic acid-rich diet in secondary prevention of coronary heart disease," *Lancet* 343 (1994): 1454–1459.

marine-derived omega-3 fatty acids EPA and DHA are used more efficiently by the body than ALA, and eating fish (and/or taking fish pills) remains the most effective way to boost your level of omega-3s. However, ALA is an equally important nutrient to include in your heart disease reversal plan. Therefore, the Prevent a Second Heart Attack plan recommends including *both* types of omega-3 fatty acids—ALA and EPA/DHA—in your daily diet. You learned the value of eating EPA and DHA in the last chapter. Now let's focus on the highly cardioprotective health benefits of eating ALA, because both forms of omega-3 fat work hand-in-hand to actively fight plaque buildup in your arteries.

WALNUTS AND FLAXSEEDS: SUPER SOURCES OF ALA

Walnuts and flaxseeds are two ancient plant foods that have sustained humans since the dawn of civilization—and both are top sources of ALA. The simplest (and tastiest) way to obtain at least 4 grams of ALA is to eat a handful of walnuts and 1½ tablespoons of ground flaxseeds every day. In so doing, you provide a strong artillery to your daily heart disease defense system.

Walnuts: Great taste, great fat, antioxidant gold mine

Walnuts stand apart from all other types of nuts for two reasons: (1) They provide the highest amount of the "vegetarian" omega-3 fatty acid, ALA, and (2) they are packed with the most plaque-fighting antioxidants relative to all other nuts. The type of antioxidant found in highest concentration in walnuts is the nonflavonoid polyphenol called ellagic acid (Figure 9.1). It may taste a bit bitter, but the *pellicle*—the thin brown skin that surrounds the walnut meat—is naturally rich in antioxidant polyphenols. Try to eat that portion as well when you eat your walnuts!

Walnuts are also naturally rich in vitamin E, the potent heart-healthy antioxidant, concentrated mostly in the nut kernel. Vitamin

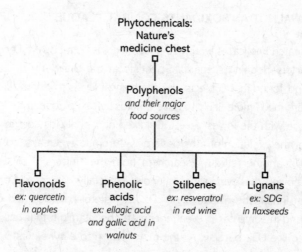

Figure 10.1. Ellagic acid and gallic acid are two powerful nonflavonoid types of polyphenol antioxidants found in high concentration in walnuts.

E is an exceptional fat-soluble vitamin because it incorporates into your LDL particle walls, strengthening them against free radical attack. More specifically, vitamin E fortifies a highly vulnerable component of the LDL wall, the phospholipid molecule, the part of the LDL particle that is particularly susceptible to oxygen's harmful effects and free-radical damage.

Flax provides ALA bonanza for your heart

Seeds from the flax plant (*Linum usitatissimum*) are ALA superstars. Flaxseeds contain the *greatest* amount of this vegetable omega-3 fatty acid of any edible plant—along with a nice dose of LDL-cholesterol-lowering soluble fiber. What's more, flaxseeds store another unique medicinal component, a type of plant hormone called *lignan*. Flax lignan, scientifically known as secoisolariciresinol diglucoside, or SDG for short, is a powerful antioxidant that can dramatically reduce plaque buildup.[1] To reap the benefits of SDG and other lignan metabolites, aim for eating the entire seed (but first be sure to grind them up—I use a coffee grinder) and not

WALNUT ANTIOXIDANTS COMBAT PLAQUE BUILDUP

New research implicates wounded phospholipids as a powerful accomplice in the artery-clogging scenario. Scientists at the University of California, San Diego, found that subjects with the highest levels of oxidized phospholipids were much more likely to have atherosclerotic plaque in their arteries than those with the lowest levels. Oxidized phospholipids contribute to all stages of the evolution of atherosclerosis—from fatty streaks to advanced plaque. In another study, researchers from the University of California, Davis, showed that walnut polyphenols, especially ellagic acid and gallic acid, can inhibit the oxidation of LDL cholesterol particles and can also protect and in some cases even regenerate the vitamin E that has incorporated into the LDL particle. All the more reason to eat walnuts, which will help strengthen your LDL particle against oxidation, *thereby preventing and reversing atherosclerosis!*

Sources: Sotirios Tsimikas et al., "Oxidized phospholipids, Lp(a) lipoprotein, and coronary artery disease," *New England Journal of Medicine* 353 (2005): 46–47; Judith A. Berliner and Andrew D. Watson, "A role for oxidized phospholipids in atherosclerosis," *New England Journal of Medicine* 353 (2005): 9–11; and Koren J. Anderson et al., "Walnut polyphenolics inhibit in vitro human plasma and LDL oxidation," *Journal of Nutrition* 131 (2001): 2837–2842.

just the flaxseed oil or a flaxseed oil supplement. That's not to say you shouldn't include flaxseed oil in your diet if you want to—after all, the oil is just another way to bump up your daily ALA intake. The reason you can't rely solely on the flaxseed oil is that it is virtually devoid of fiber, lignans, and most other nutrients (except for vitamin E) that also play an important role in heart health. (*Note:* Some flaxseed oil manufacturers do add lignans back in, so you may want to compare product labels.)

POLYUNSATURATED FATS: NOT ALL CREATED EQUALLY

You already learned that polyunsaturated fatty acids (PUFAs) are far healthier than saturated or trans fats. However, you should also know that there are two different types of essential short-chain PUFAs—alpha-linolenic acid (ALA), the omega-3 fat, and linoleic acid (LA), the omega-6 fat. Both are required by the body, yet one type is clearly the healthier choice in terms of cardioprotection. Both ALA and LA are short-chain *parent essential fatty acids*— *parent* because they spawn their respective long-chain fatty acids, and *essential* because the human body can't synthesize them, and hence we must eat them in our diet.

Omega-3 PUFAs, as you know, are found in fatty fish (the long-chain marine variety) and also are abundant in certain plant foods such as nuts, seeds, and canola oil (the short-chain vegetarian variety). The omega-6 PUFA (LA) is found in vegetable oils such as sunflower, safflower, corn, and soybean oil, as well as in many processed foods and commercial salad dressings. These two parent classes of PUFAs must be distinguished from each other, as they are metabolically and functionally separate—and have separate effects on your heart health.

Good eicosanoids, bad eicosanoids

You have the power to protect your heart by boosting the amount of anti-inflammatory chemicals the cells in your body produce—a simple task that's as easy as choosing the right fats for your plate. When it comes to eicosanoids, you truly are what you eat. There is a competition in the body for the use of the same enzymes in the chain of biochemical reactions related to your cells' creation of longer-chain fats. Whichever type of omega fat wins the enzyme competition dictates the kind of long-chain fatty acid that is produced. Your cells then metabolize the long-chain fatty acids, either arachidonic acid (AA)—derived from the parent omega-6—or EPA and DHA (derived from ALA, the parent omega-3, although the conversion rate is low) to produce hormonelike substances called *eicosanoids*.

Eicosanoids, derived from the Greek word for "twenty," are

biologically active hormonelike substances that our cells produce from either of these long-chain essential fatty acids. Eicosanoids participate in an array of bodily functions. There are "good" eicosanoids and "bad" eicosanoids.

Good eicosanoids do the following:

- Promote a relaxed dilated artery
- Reduce inflammation
- Prevent platelets from clumping together
- Promote healthy arteries

Bad eicosanoids do the following:

- Promote blood clotting
- Promote constriction of blood vessels and hardening of arteries
- Stimulate inflammation
- Promote heart disease

Hence, some eicosanoids propel the process of atherosclerosis, whereas others retard it. Your heart health is actually a function of balance between the production of the good and the bad eicosanoids, so follow the instructions in this chapter and take control of your heart health!

Manipulating your ratio of essential fatty acids

Biologically speaking, humans are wired to subsist on a diet with an omega-6 to omega-3 ratio of 1 to 1. That's what our bodies are *supposed* to get—yet the current ratio of omega-6 to omega-3 in the United States has been estimated to be as high as 17 to 1.[2] It's important to note that omega-6 isn't inherently bad—the problem is that our *proportions* are off. This imbalance (omega-6 overload coupled with an omega-3 deficiency) has severe negative health ramifications; it contributes to the development of disease because the metabolites of omega-6 fat (eicosanoids) result in inflammation. Because atherosclerosis is an inflammatory disorder, you as a heart disease patient must shift your dietary intake away from the inflammation-promoting ratio of omega-6 to omega-3 fats in your diet.

Armed with the knowledge that an unbalanced state of eicosanoid synthesis can contribute to the progression of atherosclerosis, you should use the following nutrition strategy to favorably manipulate your cell's eicosanoid production: Make a concerted effort to *eat less omega-6 fat (soybean oil, safflower oil, sunflower oil, and other vegetable oils) and more omega-3 fats (walnuts, flaxseeds, fish oil)*. In Chapter 9, we focused on the heart-health benefits of fish-derived omega-3 fats, DHA and EPA. Getting in your daily prescription (at least 4 grams) of the plant-derived omega-3 PUFA ALA can help boost your omega-3 intake, and it confers some exceptional heart benefits, too.

Flood your body with daily servings of omega-3 fats and they will incorporate into the membranes of your endothelium (the cells that form the lining of your coronary arteries). Your endothelial cells will then draw on this reserve to build the good *anti-inflammatory* eicosanoids—hormonelike substances formed within the cells from your body's metabolism of membrane-bound essential fatty acids. The healthy eicosanoids then suppress production of meddlesome adhesion molecules that sprout out from endothelial cell membranes, attracting immune cells and propagating plaque buildup.

How much is enough? The National Academy of Sciences recommends a daily ALA intake of 1.6 and 1.1 grams per day for men and women, respectively. However, to halt and reverse atherosclerosis, this recommendation is simply not high enough. Again, the best way to alter your ratio to achieve optimum health benefits is to *consume much less of the omega-6 fat LA and much more of the omega-3 fats: ALA and EPA/DHA*. It is difficult if not impossible to get in a 1-to-1 ratio, so the Prevent a Second Heart Attack plan uses the following strategy: Subtract LA from your diet by making extra virgin olive oil *your main fat* (recall that EVOO is composed of primarily super-heart-healthy monounsaturated fat, containing very little—only about 1.5%—omega-3 fat in the form of ALA), and then add in both kinds of omega-3 fats: fish oil (a small piece of fatty fish at least three times a week plus a daily 1-gram prescription fish oil supplement) and ALA (walnuts and flaxseeds, eaten daily). Note that it's not feasible or desirable in terms of maximum cardio-protection to make omega-3s your main fat. (Although omega-3 fats are phenomenal anti-inflammatory fats, they are not as stable as monounsaturated fat, which is better at protecting LDL particles from oxidation.) Aim for at least 4 grams of ALA, the plant omega-3 fat, per day. This amount of ALA can easily be obtained by eating your Prevent a Second Heart Attack daily food prescription: a handful of walnuts and 1½ tablespoons of ground flaxseeds.

Again, be sure to make your main source of fat extra virgin olive oil and avoid eating foods that are major sources of LA: safflower oil, corn oil, sunflower oil, soybean oil, cottonseed oil, sesame seed oil, brazil nuts, pine nuts, and oil-roasted nuts and seeds such as pecans and sunflower seeds. Read labels of salad dressings and pass on those with these oils. Instead, use extra virgin olive oil, balsamic vinegar, and a splash of lemon juice to dress your salads.

DAILY HEART DISEASE REVERSAL STRATEGY: WALNUTS' AND FLAXSEEDS' CONTRIBUTION

Strategy 1. Make your dysfunctional endothelium more functional

Consuming walnuts, rich in both ALA and antioxidants, will improve the functioning of your artery's endothelial layer by reducing inflammation and promoting more relaxed and dilated blood vessels.

An olive oil–rich Mediterranean diet without walnuts is not as heart-healthy as a Mediterranean diet with walnuts. Or so say a group of Spanish scientists who tested the effect of walnuts on endothelial dysfunction. Twenty-one subjects with high cholesterol were placed on one of two diets, a Mediterranean control diet (without walnuts) or a Mediterranean walnut diet, for four weeks. The walnut diet included eight to thirteen walnuts a day (between 3.7 and 6.0 grams of ALA), replacing some of the olive oil and other monounsaturated fatty acid–rich foods in the control diet. The walnut diet clearly was superior to the control diet in improving the functioning of the subjects' arteries. The daily dose of walnuts, added to an olive oil–heavy Mediterranean-style diet, resulted in a relaxation of the arteries as well as a decrease in inflammation, as evidenced by fewer adhesion molecules visible on the endothelium.[3]

One explanation for the widening of the arteries is that walnuts contain a sizable amount of an unusually artery-friendly amino acid (remember those building blocks of protein from Chapter 8?) called arginine. (Subjects on the walnut diet increased arginine intake from 0.9 to 1.4 grams per day—the amount in about a handful of walnuts.) Arginine is the precursor substance to the arterial relaxation chemical nitric oxide. Low amounts of nitric oxide and a high number of sticky adhesion molecules often characterize a dysfunctional endothelium. Therefore, walnuts' ability to relax and dilate the arteries and lessen the propensity for the diseased arterial wall to collect white blood cells makes ALA-rich walnuts a delightfully tasty and healing food to include in your heart disease reversal diet on a daily basis.

Strategy 2. Lower your cholesterol

Both walnuts and flaxseeds will work together to make a dent in your "bad" LDL cholesterol level. You learned in Chapter 2 why driving down your circulating level of LDL cholesterol is crucial for preventing another heart attack.

DO THE "TWO-STEP" TO CUT YOUR LDL DOWN TO SIZE

Not only does eating walnuts make a dent in your "bad" cholesterol, but the mere habit of snacking also contributes to lowering LDL. Snack on walnuts and you get two for one in terms of applying dietary strategies to control your cholesterol. Studies on high meal frequency (nibbling over the course of the day versus gorging on one or two meals per day) has shown that "nibbling" or increasing your meal frequency is by far the healthier habit. One study of more than two thousand men and women age fifty to eighty-nine in Rancho Bernardo, California, revealed that bumping meals up from one or two a day to four (by eating three main meals and at least one snack) can significantly cut your bad LDL cholesterol. So nibble on those walnuts as a snack and take two steps to cut your bad cholesterol down to size. But don't go too nuts for these nuts, as walnuts (like all nuts) do pack in the calories, a whopping 190 calories per ounce. Remember, a little (a handful and not a bowlful!) goes a very long way.

Source: Sharon L. Edelstein et al., "Increased meal frequency associated with decreased cholesterol concentrations; Rancho Bernardo, CA, 1984–1987," *American Journal of Clinical Nutrition* 55 (1992): 664–669.

Walnuts are effective in helping the body to rid itself of harmful LDL cholesterol, because of the ability of ALA from walnuts to incorporate itself into the wall of the LDL particles. The LDL wall becomes more flexible, which aids the liver in clearing them from the bloodstream. A recent study out of Loma Linda University in California demonstrated the value of incorporating *both* fatty fish and walnuts into your day, as each food favorably affects your blood fat profile differently. Recall that omega-3 fish fat is highly effective at lowering your blood triglyceride level, whereas consuming ALA-rich walnuts will significantly reduce your level of LDL cholesterol. Researchers recruited twenty-five healthy adults, assigning them to either a walnut diet or a fish (salmon) diet. After four weeks, the walnut group had a significant decrease in their LDL cholesterol (9.3 percent compared to the control group), whereas the fish diet led to decreased blood levels of triglycerides (11 percent compared to the control and walnut groups) as well as a 4 percent increase in their level of "good"

HDL cholesterol.[4] This reinforces the Prevent a Second Heart Attack strategy of fortifying your daily defense system by combining intake of multiple foods together (such as fish and walnuts) to attack your disease from different angles.

Flaxseeds are equally effective in lowering LDL cholesterol, and when they are eaten in combination with walnuts, their LDL-lowering effect is magnified. In one study, researchers administered 4 tablespoons of ground flaxseeds per day to postmenopausal women with moderately high LDL cholesterol. At the end of the three-month treatment period, the flaxseed group lowered their LDL cholesterol by 7 percent.[5]

Strategy 3. Make your blood less likely to clot

Research shows that ALA, once ingested, actually gets incorporated into your body's cells. What's more, it can change the physiology of your blood and make it less likely to clot. Researchers looked at blood platelets (the small fragments of cells that lead to the formation of blood clots) of two groups of young healthy men. One group was fed 40 grams per day of flaxseed oil (a rich source of ALA) and the other an equal amount of sunflower seed oil (a rich source of LA). Results showed that the flaxseed group had double the level of EPA in their platelets (derived from the conversion of ALA), which rendered the platelets much less likely to clump together and cause deadly blood clotting.[6]

Strategy 4. Lower your blood level of inflammation

We know that consumption of fish oil omega-3 fatty acids DHA and EPA is linked with lower levels of inflammation (reflected by low C-reactive protein levels, which is how doctors gauge inflammation in your blood).[7] Does the plant-derived omega-3 ALA have a similar inflammation-dampening effect? In a study designed to assess the effect of ingesting ALA on markers of inflammation (including CRP), seventy-six men with high cholesterol were placed on one of two diets: a high-ALA diet or a safflower oil diet. After three months, the men consuming the ALA diet showed a 38 percent reduction in blood CRP level, with no effect on CRP level in the safflower oil diet group.[8] This study provides clear evidence of the protective role ALA plays as an anti-inflammatory agent that will soothe the chronic inflammation that perpetuates atherosclerosis in your arteries.

TIPS FOR GETTING IN YOUR DAILY DOSE OF WALNUTS AND FLAXSEEDS

ALA IN WALNUTS AND FLAXSEEDS

Food Serving	Amount of ALA (grams)*
Walnuts, English (a.k.a. California walnuts), 1 ounce or 14 halves, approximately 190 calories	~2.6
Flaxseeds, ground, 1½ tablespoons, approximately 50 calories	~2.2

*Aim for a total daily intake of at least 4 grams.

Eating walnuts is probably the easiest and tastiest way to incorporate ALA into your day because they can be enjoyed multiple ways: as a handy and portable snack or as an embellishment to any meal. Flaxseeds, with their sweet nutty flavor, are also a delicious source of ALA and simple to fit in if you plan ahead. Here are some ideas to help you get in your daily dose of ALA:

• Keep a bag of shelled walnuts on your kitchen counter and grab some nuts as a quick and healthy snack.
• Go Greek: Enjoy a fat-free Greek yogurt (filled with the blood pressure–lowering and bone-building mineral calcium) topped with a little honey, some crushed walnuts, and ground flaxseeds, and savor a nutritious choice that makes a sensational and satisfying sweet dessert.

- Sprinkle walnuts on your green salads.

- Try candied walnuts—bake walnuts sprinkled with a little brown sugar for a sweet treat.

- Use walnuts in cooking to add taste and nutrition to your favorite dishes. You'll be surprised at how some foods truly come alive with the addition of these nuts. For example, try Chef Julie Korhumel's Basil Pesto and Tomato Whole-Wheat Crostini (made with walnuts) on page 280. Or try my spectacularly delectable, double-omega-3-whammy recipe from my previous book, *Cholesterol Down* (Three Rivers Press): Walnut-Encrusted Salmon (on page 222).

- Toss walnuts and dried fruit together in a small plastic bag and you have a super-antioxidant-rich and convenient snack for when you are out and about or even as a late-afternoon pick-me-up.

- Add ground flaxseeds to your morning oatmeal.

- Add ground flaxseeds to your pancake mix.

- Sprinkle ground flaxseeds into muffin batter or other baked goods (and you automatically cut back on the amount of fat needed in the recipe).

HEART HEALTH IN A NUTSHELL

One of the classic components of the Mediterranean eating style is that it is extremely low in "bad" fats (saturated fat, trans fat, and dietary cholesterol) and very high in "good" fats (omega-3 and monounsaturated fat). That's where walnuts and flaxseeds come in. Walnuts are packed with good fat—80 percent of their calories come from primarily omega-3 ALA (not artery-clogging saturated fat). Flaxseeds are Mother Nature's prize source of ALA. Combine the two on a daily basis and you tap into the miraculous anti-inflammatory power of plant fat to help reverse your disease.

I urge you to do your arteries a favor . . . it's high time for all

Americans to make an "oil change." Act today to cut down on those pro-inflammatory omega-6 fats while simultaneously making a conscious effort to increase your intake of ultra-heart-healthy ALA omega-3s, and you will be taking some powerful steps to stop atherosclerosis in its tracks.

Heart-Healthy Food Number 7: Oatmeal and Other Whole Grains

Man is what he eats.

—Ludwig Andreas von Feuerbach, German philosopher and anthropologist
(1804–1872)

 Eat oatmeal and other whole grains every day.

Companion foods Rx: at least three servings (48 grams) of whole grains every day:

- Complete whole grains such as oatmeal, barley, corn, popcorn, brown rice, quinoa, or bulgur wheat
- Foods with added whole grains such as 100 percent whole-grain breads or cereals, whole-wheat pasta, or foods with added whole-wheat flour

Primary disease-fighting bioactive compounds:

- Polyphenol antioxidants: avenanthramides (oats)
- Polyphenol phenolic acids: ferulic acid and caffeic acid
- Soluble fiber (beta-glucan) and insoluble fiber
- Antioxidant vitamin: vitamin E
- Antioxidant mineral: selenium

OATMEAL: HEART HEALTH IN A BOWL

You've heard it before: Oatmeal protects the heart. And rest assured, the man on the Quaker oatmeal box isn't lying—oatmeal is a whole grain, a type of plant food and complex carbohydrate that makes up the backbone of the heart-healthiest Mediterranean style of eating. Choosing whole grains as your main form of carbohydrate nourishment has been scientifically proven to thwart heart disease, cutting the risk of coronary artery disease by a phenomenal 40 percent.[1] In fact, consuming 2.5 servings of whole grains a day has been shown to lower the risk of a cardiac event by 21 percent compared to eating less than one serving a day.[2] In terms of preventing a second heart attack, going for the (whole) grain is a key feature of the Prevent a Second Heart Attack plan, because whole-grain intake *can halt the progression of atherosclerosis* in individuals already diagnosed with coronary artery disease.[3]

Whole grains are a virtual medicine chest filled with plant nutrients, antioxidants, vitamins, minerals, and fiber that when combined with your daily legume prescription provide you with all the amino acids your body needs for good health, and in just the right proportions. All the bioactive compounds in whole grains work together to keep your heart and blood vessels healthy, and oatmeal is a stellar grain that stands out among the whole-grain crowd.

A morning bowl of oatmeal delivers plaque-fighting, nutrient-dense benefits that last all day. Oats are an energy-yielding complex carbohydrate that keeps you fuller longer, by slowly releasing glucose into your bloodstream. Moreover, oats house a rare type of soluble fiber called beta-glucan, a highly effective LDL-lowering substance. Oats are king when it comes to soluble fiber, having the highest proportion of any grain. They also contain insoluble fiber, which benefits your digestive health.

Oats are unique among grains because they come packaged with their own special plaque-busting antioxidant polyphenols called avenanthramides. Avenanthramides work magic on your endothelium, which may be one reason for oats' super-heart-healthy status. Recall from Chapter 2 that the intimal layer of healthy blood vessel walls contains relatively few smooth muscle cells. However, in damaged vessels, and as fatty streaks evolve into the more dangerous plaque, smooth muscle cells migrate into the intima and

---

SCIENCE BACKING OATS' HEART BENEFITS STRONGER THAN EVER

Oats made health food history when in 1997 they were the first food to garner a coveted U.S. Food and Drug Administration (FDA) health claim. The FDA allowed this claim based on a large collection of scientific evidence showing that consumption of whole-oat sources of soluble fiber reduces blood cholesterol. An up-to-date review of the science backing oats for heart health published in the *American Journal of Lifestyle Medicine* supports the FDA's decades-old conclusion. New insight into oats' spectacular cardioprotective properties includes, in addition to LDL lowering, favorable changes in LDL physical characteristics (i.e., making them fatter and fluffier), as well as making LDL less susceptible to oxidation. Regular oat consumption has also been shown to reduce risk of high blood pressure, weight gain, and type 2 diabetes.

Sources: U.S Department of Human Services, Federal Register 62 FR 15343, "Food labeling: Health claims; Soluble fiber from oats and risk of coronary artery disease; Final rule, March 31, 1997," http://www.fda.gov/Food/LabelingNutrition/LabelClaims/HealthClaimsMeetingSignificantScientific AgreementSSA/ucm074514.htm; and Mark B. Andon and James W. Anderson, "State of the art reviews: The oatmeal-cholesterol connection 10 years later," *American Journal of Lifestyle Medicine* 2, no. 1 (2008): 51–57.

reproduce. This migration and multiplication of smooth muscle cells within the arterial wall is a major contributing factor to the progression of atherosclerosis. Scientists have shown that avenanthramides can stop the proliferation of smooth muscle cells in their tracks, thus derailing a key course of action in plaque progression.[4]

ROUGH UP YOUR DIET TO SAVE YOUR HEART

Are you, like so many Americans, fearful of eating carbs because you think they're fattening? That's unfortunate, because if you cut back on carbs, and especially the "good" carbs, you automatically reduce your intake of the top dietary source of fiber. The government recommends that we make at least half of our daily grains whole (which comes to at least three servings of whole grains per day), but most Americans—96 percent—fall short of that goal. The truth is, most Americans fail to get in even one serving of whole grains per day.[5] This is a problem because whole grains are a high-fiber food, and high-fiber diets prevent a host of conditions including heart disease, certain types of cancer, obesity, and may even extend life.

How much fiber should you eat?

A pooled analysis of ten U.S. and European studies providing a very large scientific database (more than 2.5 million men and women) found that every 10-gram increase in daily intake of cereal fiber reduces the risk of a coronary event by 10 percent and the risk of death from heart disease by 25 percent.[6] Just how much fiber should you be eating for good health? According to the recommendations from the Institute of Medicine's Food and Nutrition Board, men and women age fifty and younger should consume 38 grams and 25 grams, respectively, of dietary fiber per day. (An example of foods that add up to about 38 grams of fiber would be 1 bowl of oatmeal (4 grams), 1 tablespoon of ground flaxseeds

(3 grams), 1 cup of blackberries (7 grams), 1 cup of cooked lentils (15 grams) served over 1 cup of brown rice (3 grams), 1 cup of cooked spinach (4 grams), and 1 ounce of walnuts (2 grams). Men and women older than fifty have a lower recommendation at 30 grams and 21 grams per day, respectively.[7] Unfortunately, our dietary intake falls woefully short of these recommendations. The American Heart Association estimates that the average American eats just 15 grams of dietary fiber per day or about half the amount your body needs.

Perhaps we should all listen to the generations of grandmothers who were wise enough to have lobbied for diets rich in whole grains, fruits, and vegetables because of their "roughage." The easiest way to bump up your fiber intake is to ingest plenty of good

---

POPCORN: A WHOLE-GRAIN AND FIBER GOLD MINE

Who knew? Corn, the tiny kernel that most of the world calls maize (after the Spanish word *maíz*), is a bona fide whole grain, and yes, even the popped version counts. People who routinely snack on popcorn ingest a whopping 250 percent more whole grains and 22 percent more fiber compared to those who don't eat this dieter's delight. (Popcorn contains more fiber per ounce than even whole-wheat bread and brown rice.) Researchers evaluated dietary intake information from the 1999–2002 National Health and Nutrition Examination Survey, a large government-run program designed to assess the health and nutritional status of Americans. The findings? People who routinely snacked on popcorn were way ahead of the game in terms of their whole-grain and fiber intake. (Five cups of air-popped popcorn provides you with 5 grams of dietary fiber and 40 grams of whole grains, and all for a mere 150 calories.) So snack away, but just be sure to avoid the unhealthy additives, butter and salt, that ruin a perfectly heart-healthy food.

Source: Ann C. Grandjean et al., "Popcorn consumption and dietary and physiological parameters of US children and adults: Analysis of the National Health and Nutrition Examination Survey (NHANES) 1999–2002 dietary survey data," *Journal of the American Dietetic Association* 108, no. 5 (2008): 853–856.

carbs and follow the plant-based eating strategy (fruits, vegetables, legumes, walnuts, and whole grains) espoused in the Prevent a Second Heart Attack plan. But fiber isn't the only good thing to come out of eating whole grains. Fiber is only one part of the whole (grain) picture, and in this case, the whole is truly greater than the sum of its parts. Read on and see what other healing components are encapsulated within these small but mighty kernels of grain.

WHAT MAKES WHOLE GRAINS "WHOLE"?

What's the real difference between white rice and brown? Choose the white variety and you swallow a fiberless bundle of starch—fortified with iron and some B vitamins, but still missing many key nutrients located in the *bran,* the outer fibrous layer covering the rice kernel that has been removed during refining. Choose the brown rice and you will be eating a grain the way Mother Nature packaged it, a wonderful source of an array of natural vitamins and minerals, antioxidants, and fiber—nutrients that are mostly lost in the refining process.

Whole grains' three-part package

Natural whole grains contain three botanically defined parts: the bran, the endosperm, and the germ (or embryo). Eat the whole seed, or *kernel,* with the three parts intact—the entire complex—and you are eating a complete whole grain that packs a powerful nutritional punch.

• The *bran* is the multilayered outer skin of the kernel. Most of the healthy disease-fighting phytochemicals are concentrated in the bran layer, as are most of the minerals and fiber.

• The *endosperm* is the energy-containing center, largely starch, that is the germ's food supply.

• The *germ* resides inside the endosperm; it is the nutrient storehouse, containing healthy fats, vitamins, minerals, and some protein.

Whole grains contain all three parts of the kernel. Refined grains have had the bran and most of the germ portions removed, so you are basically left eating just the endosperm of the rice kernel when you choose white rice over brown. When you remove the germ and bran layers, you lose most of the fiber, B vitamins, vitamin E, and healthy fats, and about 75 percent of the phytochemicals and antioxidants.[8] Thus, when you eliminate these parts of the kernel in processing, you strip the grain of much of its disease-fighting potential. In fact, refining wheat, another type of grain, removes most of the naturally occurring vitamins, minerals, and other nutrients, including the lion's share of wheat's potent polyphenol antioxidant, ferulic acid.[9]

FAIL TO EAT WHOLE-GRAIN BREAKFAST CEREAL AND YOUR HEART COULD FAIL

Heart failure (a.k.a. congestive heart failure) occurs when the heart becomes less efficient at pumping blood to the rest of the body. It is a life-threatening condition and the leading cause of hospitalizations for older Americans (the prognosis remains poor because drug treatment is only partially effective). Heart failure often develops as the result of clogged arteries and is common among people who have had a previous heart attack. The good news is that a recent study confirms that the simple habit of eating a whole-grain cereal for breakfast every day can cut your risk of heart failure.

Harvard researchers decided to investigate the effects of cereal consumption on heart failure risk in a study involving roughly 21,000 male doctors with an average age of fifty-four years who were followed for nearly twenty years. It was found that men who ate a bowl of whole-grain cereal a day had an impressive 29 percent reduced risk of heart failure!

Sources: U.S. National Library of Medicine and the National Institutes of Health, "Heart failure," http://www.nlm.nih.gov/medlineplus/ency/article/000158.htm; and Luc Djoussé and Michael Gaziano, "Breakfast cereal and risk of heart failure in the Physicians' Health Study I," *Archives of Internal Medicine* 167, no. 19 (2007): 2080–2085.

IDENTIFYING WHOLE-GRAIN PRODUCTS
AT THE SUPERMARKET

Walk down the bread aisle and you are bombarded with products boasting *multigrain, wheat fiber, high fiber,* and *whole wheat.* How can you be sure that the product you choose contains the real McCoy, a full serving or more of whole grains? (*Note:* Foods claiming to be "whole grain" come in one of two varieties—either as *a complete whole grain in a single food,* such as brown rice or popcorn, or as *an ingredient in a multi-ingredient food,* such as whole-wheat flour in bread, or millet or buckwheat groats in cereal.) To avoid confusion, aim for eating lots of whole-grain single foods and be judicious about reading labels for multi-ingredient foods. Look for the FDA seal of approval to ensure that the product is indeed whole grain. In 1999, the FDA endorsed a health claim for whole-grain foods: "Diets rich in whole-grain foods and other plant foods, and low in total fat, saturated fat and cholesterol, may reduce the risk of heart disease and certain cancers."[10] If the food bears this FDA whole-grain health claim, you are guaranteed that the product contains 51 percent or more whole grains by weight.

You can also look for the Whole Grains Council's "stamps" on certain foods. The Whole Grains Council is a nonprofit consumer advocacy group dedicated to promoting greater consumption of whole grains to improve health. It places its packaging symbol on products that are guaranteed to contain whole grains. Two types of stamps are allowed on food products: the basic stamp and the 100 percent stamp. The basic stamp means that the grains in the product may contain refined grains in addition to whole grains and that one serving of the food has at least a half serving of whole grains. The 100 percent stamp means that one serving of the food contains a serving or more of whole—and only whole—grains. The obvious choice is foods with the 100 percent stamp.

If the product does not bear either the FDA claim or the 100

"WHOLE" LINGO TO LOOK FOR IN THE INGREDIENT LIST

Words that signify whole grains:

- The word *whole* listed before a grain, such as "whole rye flour"
- The term *100% whole wheat*
- The words *berries* or *groats,* such as "wheat berries" or "oat groats"
- The words *rolled oats* and *oatmeal*
- *Brown rice* and *wild rice*

Misleading terms:

- The words *wheat flour, refined enriched flour,* and *unbleached wheat flour* do not indicate whole grains.
- Graham flour is a whole grain, but graham crackers do not have to be predominantly whole grain, because they are usually made with mostly *enriched wheat flour.*
- *100% wheat, multigrain,* and the phrase *contains whole grain*

Source: U.S. Department of Agriculture, "HealthierUS School Challenge: Whole grains resource," http://www.fns.usda.gov/tn/healthierus/wholegrainresource.pdf.

---

percent stamp, turn the package over and check the Nutrition Facts panel. Zero in on the ingredients list and look for the word *whole* before the grain's name. Prepared foods should ideally have the whole grain as the first ingredient listed, such as brown rice, whole-wheat flour, or whole corn. It is always a wiser nutrition choice to select whole, unprocessed grain products compared to the refined, processed varieties such as corn flakes or white bread.

Going for the (whole) grain

To help you fill your Prevent a Second Heart Attack plan whole-grain prescription, consult the following list and make sure you get in at least three whole-grain servings per day for a total of at least 48 grams.

Amaranth: a traditional food grain in Africa, with approximately 30 percent higher protein content than cereals

Barley: whole barley, whole barley flour, whole-grain barley, dehulled barley

Buckwheat, including buckwheat groats and whole buckwheat flour

Corn, whole corn and corn flour, popcorn, whole-grain cornmeal

Millet, including millet flour

Oats: whole oats, oat groats, rolled oats, oatmeal, whole-oat flour

Quinoa, including quinoa flour

Rice: brown rice, brown rice flour, wild rice, wild rice flour

Rye: whole rye, whole rye flour, rye berries

Sorghum (milo): a staple whole-grain source of nutrition in India

Teff: an ancient whole-grain cereal crop commonly grown in Ethiopia

Triticale: a tasty hybrid of wheat and rye, originally bred in Scotland and Sweden

Wheat: whole-wheat flour, cracked wheat, spelt, emmer, farro, durum, kamut, bulgur (cracked wheat), crushed wheat, sprouted wheat, wheat berries, graham flour (coarsely ground whole-wheat flour), whole white-wheat flour

DAILY HEART DISEASE REVERSAL STRATEGY: WHOLE GRAINS' CONTRIBUTION

Strategy 1. Boost total antioxidant capacity and curb LDL oxidation

Getting in your daily whole-grain prescription will raise your blood's total antioxidant capacity (TAC) because whole grains are virtual antioxidant factories, housing a nice amount of vitamin E, the mineral selenium, and the polyphenol phenolic acids ferulic acid and caffeic acid.

Most people are unaware that whole grains possess strong disease-fighting antioxidant activity. In fact, the average antioxidant activity of whole grains is actually *greater* than that of most fruits and vegetables.[11] Remember, the antioxidants and other phyto-chemicals are most concentrated in the bran and the germ of the kernel—so make sure you're eating the *whole* oat or grain, not its refined counterpart.[12] If you miss out on any part of the grain—the bran, for example—you could miss out on as much as 98 percent of those TAC-enhancing antioxidants.

A last note on TAC: Remember to eat your grains *throughout* the day, in order to maintain a high level of antioxidants in your bloodstream and build up your antioxidant defense system 24/7.

Strategy 2. Stabilize vulnerable plaque by lowering LDL cholesterol

Eating your whole grains, especially oats and barley, will make a sig-nificant dent in your LDL cholesterol, reducing it an average of 14 mg/dL for oats and 10 mg/dL for barley.[13] Many of the foods and the exercise promoted in the Prevent a Second Heart Attack plan work in unison to lower your LDL cholesterol. Combine this lifestyle approach with your physician-prescribed statin medication and you have a complete, intensive LDL-lowering therapy for con-trolling your disease—recall from Chapter 1 the tremendous im-portance of getting that LDL down to less than 70 mg/dL.

Strategy 3. Prevent and treat high blood pressure

Eating whole grains can slash your risk of developing high blood pressure, another factor that significantly increases your risk of hav-ing a second attack. That's the news from the most recent results of the ongoing Health Professionals Follow-Up Study, begun in 1986, in which more than 51,000 male health professionals con-tinue to provide health data and detailed dietary information at four-year intervals. This particular subset followed 33,000 men, without high blood pressure at the onset, for eighteen years, during which their diet and lifestyle habits as well as health status were tracked. According to Harvard researchers, the men who had the highest intake of whole grains (bran in particular), estimated at 46 grams of whole grains per day, had a 19 percent reduced risk of developing high blood pressure compared to men who consumed just 3 grams of whole grains a day.[14]

If you already have high blood pressure, the simple act of swapping brown rice for white, 100 percent whole-grain bread for white bread, and barley for refined grains can lower your blood pressure a statistically measurable amount after just five weeks.[15]

Strategy 4. Prevent and treat metabolic syndrome and type 2 diabetes

Eating whole grains will lessen your risk of contracting metabolic syndrome—the constellation of metabolic disturbances that predisposes you to developing type 2 diabetes and accelerates atherosclerosis.[16] If you have already been diagnosed with metabolic syndrome, take heart in knowing that eating whole grains will improve your blood sugar metabolism and can delay or prevent the progression of metabolic syndrome to type 2 diabetes.[17]

Whole grains, and especially whole grains containing a large cache of the LDL-draining soluble fiber beta-glucan (found in high concentration in oats, barley, and rye), are particularly helpful in treating blood sugar abnormalities. The gel-forming property of the soluble type of fiber in the intestines is responsible for regulating your circulating blood sugar level. Beta-glucan is beneficial for controlling blood sugar because it acts like a sponge, trapping carbohydrates and thereby delaying their release from the stomach into the intestines as well as slowing the absorption of carbohydrates into the bloodstream.

Insulin resistance is the body's inability to control its blood

---

WHOLE-GRAIN MEDITERRANEAN DIET STAVES OFF NEED FOR DRUGS IN PEOPLE NEWLY DIAGNOSED WITH DIABETES

Italian research published in 2009 involving more than two hundred people newly diagnosed with type 2 diabetes compared a traditional American Heart Association low-fat diet with a whole-grain-rich, moderate-carbohydrate Mediterranean diet. After four years, people on the Mediterranean diet lost more weight and needed less medication to treat their diabetes. Only 44 percent of the participants who stuck with the Mediterranean diet required blood-sugar-lowering medication compared to 70 percent of people on the low-fat diet. According to the researchers, the whole-grain-rich Mediterranean diet was clearly the superior dietary treatment for people with type 2 diabetes. What did the diet consist of? Carbohydrate intake was mostly in the form of whole grains, nuts, fruits, and vegetables, capped at up to 50 percent of daily calories. Compared to the low-fat diet, it included fewer carbs and a much larger amount of the "healthy" fat, olive oil (used as the subjects' main fat).

Source: Katherine Esposito et al., "Effects of a Mediterranean-style diet on the need for antihyperglycemic drug therapy in patients with newly diagnosed type 2 diabetes: A randomized trial," *Annals of Internal Medicine* 151, no. 5 (2009): 306–314.

---

sugar level with a normal level of insulin and an early step in the development of type 2 diabetes. Whole grains can make insulin-resistant muscles, well, less resistant. In 2003, the results of a study examining the relationship between whole-grain intake and the development of metabolic disorders and diabetes was published in the *American Journal of Clinical Nutrition*. Whole-grain eaters were found to have a lower fasting insulin blood concentration (called *improved insulin sensitivity*) when compared to individuals who subsisted on mostly refined grains. Thus, the researchers concluded that whole grains have an "insulin-sensitizing" method of action in the body.[18]

Eating whole grains can have a dramatic effect on your odds of developing type 2 diabetes, a disease you want to aggressively prevent or manage because 75 percent of people with diabetes will die from heart disease. Findings from a meta-analysis of six studies examining the relationship between whole-grain consumption and the development of type 2 diabetes found that for each two-servings-per-day increment in whole-grain intake, risk of type 2 diabetes dropped 21 percent.[19]

Strategy 5. Control your weight and prevent obesity

Filling your daily whole-grain prescription will help you control your weight, which is important because being overweight or obese is an independent risk factor for heart disease. In another subset of the Health Professionals Follow-Up Study, a group of more than 27,000 healthy men at the onset was followed for eight years to examine the potential association between whole-grain intake and long-term weight gain. The researchers calculated each subject's whole-grain intake (in grams) per day. Those who ate the most whole grains were leaner at the end of the eight-year reporting period. Specifically, weight gain was reduced by approximately 2.5 pounds for each 40-gram increment in daily whole-grain intake—an amount equal to about two slices of 100 percent whole-grain bread. The researchers concluded that the high fiber and high water content of whole grains lessened weight gain by promoting satiety. Whole-grain foods also contain fewer calories than the equivalent weight of a refined grain.[20]

TIPS FOR GETTING IN YOUR DAILY DOSE OF WHOLE GRAINS

• Make oatmeal your breakfast of choice on most days of the week. Cook up a large batch of the steel-cut version, which is highest in beta-glucan. Steel-cut oatmeal takes longer to cook but is well worth it for the superior taste, texture, and health benefits. Keep a large stash of cooked oatmeal in the refrigerator (in a sealed container), then portion it out and heat daily servings for a heart-disease-reversing breakfast in minutes.

• Substitute 100 percent whole-wheat toast for bagels and 100 percent whole-grain muffins for pastries. Make all your sandwiches with 100 percent whole-grain bread or pita.

• Have a slice of veggie pizza made with whole-grain crust for lunch.

• Be adventurous and expand your grain repertoire with interesting new tastes such as amaranth, quinoa, and spelt.

• Snack on popcorn, a tasty and filling snack that's good for your heart and your waistline. Nix the theater popcorn or microwave bags and pull out the antique hot-air popper, or better yet, pop the kernels in a brown paper lunch bag in the microwave. Season with a few sprays of olive oil and a touch of Parmesan cheese or brown sugar—depending on whether you crave salty or sweet.

• Try a recipe with barley, a delightfully tasty and wholesome grain that contains all the cholesterol-lowering heart-healthy ingredients of oatmeal. Perhaps a barley risotto, barley added to stew or salad, a barley pilaf, or a comforting barley soup on a cold winter's day.

QUINOA: THE MOTHER OF ALL GRAINS

Quinoa (KEEN-wah) is one of those "ancient" grains that is actually not native to the Mediterranean but rather South America. Quinoa was called the "mother of all grains" by the Incas, who considered it a sacred food. Quinoa is the seed of the goosefoot plant, a plant related to spinach, with leaves that resemble . . . you guessed it, the foot of a goose! Loaded with vitamins, minerals, antioxidants, and fiber, this whole grain is incredibly nutritious. Quinoa is also unique among grains because it is a complete protein, meaning it contains the right amount of all essential amino acids your body needs to build new proteins. Quinoa has twice the protein of regular cereal grains. Be adventurous and give this ancient grain a try! It has a sweet, nutty flavor with just a touch of crunch. Serve quinoa as a substitute for rice (it cooks much quicker and comes out light and fluffy) or even in salads. Most grocery stores now carry it in the rice and beans aisle.

• For dinner, try delicious wild rice as a side dish (see the wild rice side dish recipe, page 313) or a side of brown rice and some 100 percent whole-grain Italian bread (dipped in extra virgin olive oil, of course!).

• When you eat out, finding whole grains presents a bigger challenge, because few restaurants offer whole grains on the menu. Look for oatmeal or buckwheat pancakes at breakfast establishments, whole-wheat pita sandwiches at lunch, or soups made with barley. Some Asian restaurants offer a brown rice option, Italian restaurants are providing a whole-grain pasta choice, and ethnic Middle Eastern establishments offer tabouli, made with whole-grain bulgur wheat.

MAKE HEARTY WHOLE GRAINS THE STAFF OF YOUR LIFE

Hearty, healthy, whole-grain good carbs—they can cut your risk of another heart attack, lower your blood pressure, prevent diabetes, and even help you lose weight. Going Mediterranean means routinely choosing "brown" foods and avoiding the "whites"—flour, rice, and bread—opting for whole and unprocessed over refined. Whole grains are a three-part nutrient-dense package, filled with biologically active components that protect your cardiovascular system, whereas nutritionally inferior refined grains offer no such protection.

Make an effort to fill your daily prescription of at least three servings (and preferably more) of whole grains by starting your day with a delicious and nutritious bowl of steaming oatmeal, followed by other whole grains such as barley, rye, millet, and whole wheat. This dietary maneuver is one of the healthiest choices you can make, delivering your body some of Mother Nature's gold-star plant foods—rich sources of biologically active nutrients that work together to heal your damaged heart.

12

Heart-Healthy Food Number 8: Pinot Noir and Other Red Wine

During meals drink wine happily, little but often.

—Arnoldo da Villanova, Spanish alchemist and physician (1253–1315)

 Drink one to two glasses of red wine with a meal—every day.

Primary disease-fighting bioactive compounds:

- Ethanol (alcohol)
- Polyphenol antioxidant flavonoids: flavan-3-ols (procyanidins), flavonols (quercetin), anthocyanins (malvidin)
- Phenolic acids: gallic acid, caffeic acid
- Stilbene polyphenol: resveratrol

Why is it that the French routinely indulge in artery-clogging cream sauces, butter, foie gras, and other fatty, cholesterol-laden foods yet have only half the rate of heart disease that we do? The secret behind this mystery, dubbed the "French paradox" by scientists in the early 1990s, is thought to be all the red wine the French drink with their food. Something in the red wine neutralizes heart attack risk, and that something is the powerful antioxidant polyphenols. Much of the media's attention has focused on one antioxidant in particular—resveratrol, a strong stilbene polyphenol antioxidant that grapes produce on the vine in response to fungal infections and other invading pathogens. Resveratrol is found only in the skin of the grape. Because red wine is made by fermenting the juice of the fruit with the pulp—both skin and seeds—and white wine is made via fermentation of the juice alone, red wine contains resveratrol whereas white has a negligible amount.

WINE: THE DRINK OF THE AGES

Wine has been part of human culture for millennia, with evidence of wine vessels dating back seven thousand years unearthed at a Neolithic village site in Iran.[1] Wine is aptly referred to as "the drink of the ages," and wine lore permeates our world's cultures, be it in myth or medicine, passages in the Bible, or places of honor at modern social occasions. Wine has played a major role in the culture and diet of the traditional Mediterranean people, and some scientists think it is the single ingredient most responsible for the good health enjoyed by those who inhabit this area of the world.

ALCOHOL, ESPECIALLY RED WINE, IS GOOD FOR THE HEART

Without question, the scientific data is clear: Drinking alcohol regularly, and lightly to moderately with meals, guards against heart disease and lengthens life, whereas consuming high doses harms the heart and causes disease. Just how protective is sensible drinking? A strong body of scientific evidence estimates that in both men and women, light to moderate alcohol consumption reduces risk of death from a heart attack by 30 to 50 percent.[2] Although all types of alcoholic drinks (taken daily and in small amounts) are associated with a lower risk of heart disease, red wine offers the greatest cardioprotection,[3] hence the inclusion of red wine as the Prevent a Second Heart Attack plan's alcoholic beverage prescription.

Moderation is key

Drinking alcohol is clearly a case of a double-edged sword. One fact is certain: Moderation is the magic word, meaning a little is good, and a lot is *not* better. Wine is beneficial for your health *only in moderation*. But what is the definition of *moderation?* According to the U.S. Department of Health and Human Services and the U.S. Department of Agriculture, a moderate amount of red wine is defined as no more than 14 grams per day of ethanol (the equivalent of one 5-ounce glass of wine, or 150 mL) for women and no more than 28 grams per day (two glasses of wine) for men.[4]

Overdrinking can severely damage health and is associated with a sharp *increase* in risk of heart disease, high blood pressure, stroke, certain forms of cancer, liver cirrhosis, and alcohol abuse and alcoholism. Excessive drinking can also shorten your life span. So keep in mind that when it comes to your red wine consumption, the difference between drinking in moderation and drinking in excess is the difference between preventing disease and causing disease. *Include the red wine prescription in your Prevent a Second Heart Attack plan only if you and your personal physician mutually agree that you can drink safely.* And never drink and drive.

If you don't currently drink, should you start?

New research shows that even middle-aged teetotalers can garner significant heart health benefits from beginning to consume wine in moderation. The Atherosclero-

---

RED FLAG WARNINGS

- Alcohol can interact with prescription medications.
- For women at risk of breast cancer, *any amount of alcohol increases risk.*
- For pregnant women, there is no safe level of alcohol consumption.
- Avoid alcohol if you have been diagnosed with cardiomyopathy or cardiac arrhythmias.

sis Risk in Communities (ARIC) study is a ten-year prospective study of almost sixteen thousand middle-aged men and women, designed to investigate the origin and progression of atherosclerotic disease. Of the nearly 7,700 subjects who were healthy nondrinkers at the outset, after a four-year follow-up period the new adopters of moderate wine consumption cut their risk of experiencing a cardiac event by 38 percent compared to their nondrinking counterparts.[5] *Moderation* in this case was defined as one to fourteen drinks per week for men and one to seven drinks per week for women.

UNCORKING RED WINE'S HEART BENEFITS

Red wine's one-two punch against atherosclerosis

There's no question that a little wine with food can do a heart good. The best known cardioprotective effect of red wine is its ability to increase the "good" HDL cholesterol level—one to two drinks per day is linked to an average 12 percent increase in HDL.[6] The biological basis for red wine's preventive effects lies in its anti-inflammatory actions as well as its ability to positively affect the endothelial layer (the inner layer) of your arteries and reduce LDL oxidation. What exactly in this fermented grape juice is responsible for these heart health rewards? The beneficial effects of light to moderate wine drinking against atherosclerosis have been attributed to two main ingredients in red wine: the alcohol (ethanol) content and the antioxidant activity of its polyphenols.

Choose red for a super shot of plant polyphenols

Why is red wine superior to other types of alcoholic beverages such as beer or spirits? All types of alcoholic drinks contain ethanol (alcohol), and ethanol is known to have a sedative-like effect on blood vessels, causing them to relax and dilate, which increases coronary blood flow and is, as you know, a healthy state. What sets red wine apart from other drinks is that in addition to ethanol, red wine contains a complex mixture of potent plant polyphenols, many of which are responsible for the deep red garnet color of fine red wines—an outstanding heart-disease-reversing antioxidant arsenal that other alcoholic beverages simply do not contain. Ethanol is

PINOT NOIR, EXPENSIVE CABS, AND TANNAT REDS DELIVER HIGHEST POLYPHENOL CONTENT

Most of the polyphenol antioxidants in red wine are derived from the flavonoid flavon-3-ols (and more specifically the procyanidins such as catechin) and the flavonols (such as quercetin). The amount of these flavonoids varies depending on the climate and variety of grape. Pinot noir, Cabernet Sauvignon, and Tannat contain the highest levels. Flavonoid content is influenced by how much sun the grape skin receives—greater sun exposure enhances production.

Pinot noir tends to have maximum sun exposure, hence the higher level of flavonoids. To obtain the maximum flavonoid polyphenols in your Cab, you will have to pay more. One study found that luxury bottles of Cabernet Sauvignon, the kind of wine that comes from lower-yielding vines with better sun exposure, have significantly higher levels of flavonols compared to less expensive, widely sold Cabernets. Additional research has shown that the Tannat variety of red wine (made from the Tannat red wine grape) beats them all when it comes to flavonoid polyphenol content. Tannat grapes, historically grown in southwest France, have now become the "national grape" of Uruguay, and plantings in California are becoming increasingly popular.

Pinot noir has also been shown to have the highest level of the potent non-flavonoid antioxidant resveratrol. This is especially true for varieties grown in cooler, rainy locales because grapes produce resveratrol to ward off fungal infections and other environmental stresses that are more prevalent in cold, wet environments.

Sources: Andrew L. Waterhouse, "Wine phenolics," *Annals of the New York Academy of Science* 957 (2002): 21–36; Jeffrey G. Ritchey and Andrew L. Waterhouse, "A standard red wine: Monomeric phenolic analysis of commercial cabernet sauvignon," *American Journal of Enology and Viticulture* 50 (1999): 91–100; and Fernanda A. Pimentel et al., "Chocolate and red wine—A comparison between flavonoids content," *Food Chemistry* 120 (2010): 109–112.

even more beneficial when it's packaged together with polyphenols, because the combination helps increase intestinal absorption and bioavailability of the plant antioxidants.[7]

Red wine is one of the richest food sources of polyphenols. A highly tannic red wine contains more than 3 grams of total polyphenols in a liter.[8] These antioxidants mop up excess free radicals that attack the LDL particles—a key initiating event in plaque buildup. Red wine polyphenols have also been shown to partner with vitamin E to reactivate or recycle this valuable antioxidant vitamin. This is important, because vitamin E is incorporated within the LDL particle, shielding it from damage, the first line of defense against oxidation.[9]

Red wine's wide array of polyphenols can be divided into two

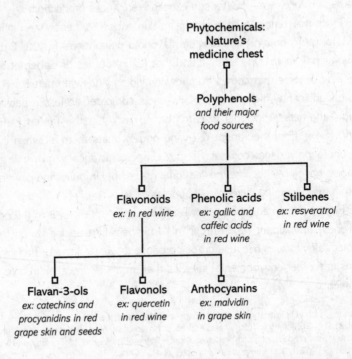

Figure 12.1: Red wine contains primarily the polyphenol flavonoids (flavan-3-ols, flavonols, and anthocyanins) and the nonflavonoids (stilbenes and phenolic acids).

main groups: (1) the nonflavonoids (stilbenes and phenolic acids) and (2) the flavonoids (flavan-3-ols, flavonols, and anthocyanins [Figure 12.1]).[10] Three specific types of polyphenols stand out among the red wine crowd for their notable cardioprotective benefits: resveratrol, procyanidins, and quercetin.

To tap into wine's huge cache of powerful polyphenols, be sure to pick red over white. Red wine has ten times the polyphenol content of white wine, because red wine is produced by fermentation of grape juice in the presence of the pulp (skins and seeds), where the polyphenols are produced. (White wine is made by quickly pressing the juice away from the grape solids; hence white wine is merely fermented fruit juice.)

Cheers to a longer life!

Although excessive drinking of alcohol can severely damage health and shorten life, moderate consumption, especially of red wine, protects against early mortality. The Mediterranean diet, in particular, has been linked to longevity. In previous chapters, you read about the Greek segment of the European Prospective Investigation into Cancer and Nutrition (EPIC) study, in which researchers from the University of Athens in Greece and the Harvard School of Public Health in Boston tried to pinpoint the ingredient in the traditional Mediterranean diet that is most responsible for prolonging life. The scientists performed a sophisticated statistical analysis to determine the relative contribution to longevity that each of the main dietary components in the diet makes. It turns out that moderate wine consumption with meals is number one, accounting for 24 percent of the benefit. Yes, you heard me right—according to this study, moderate wine drinking is the most important ingredient of the Mediterranean lifestyle in the recipe for a longer life. But before you uncork your magnum of champagne, remember— moderate, in this case, is defined as one to five small glasses of alcohol (10–50 grams of alcohol) daily for men and half that for women, mostly in the form of red wine with meals.[11] (Obviously, the definition of *moderate* differs across the pond, so to play it safe, I would suggest sticking to the maximum of one glass daily for women and two glasses for men suggested in the Prevent a Second Heart Attack plan.)

Just how much can a daily tipple increase your odds of living a long life? A recent meta-analysis of thirty-four studies involving more than one million men and women says that indeed, regularly imbibing low doses of alcohol will extend your life. Statistically speaking, a low level of alcohol intake (defined in this case as one to two drinks per day for women and two to four for men) boosts survival rate by 18 percent. Note that this study also confirmed the hazards of heavy drinking, with higher doses of alcohol associated with a hefty increase in rates of death.[12]

Fountain of youth . . . in mice and men. Resveratrol has been on the public's radar lately because of research performed on mice, linking large doses of resveratrol to an increased life span. Harvard scientists have shown that feeding resveratrol to mice can stimulate the synthesis of proteins called sirtuins that retard aging. The problem is in the translation. To attain the longevity benefits observed in mice, humans would have to drink 100 to 1,000 bottles of red wine per day to receive a resveratrol dosage equal to what was administered to the mice.

Although resveratrol has received the most attention and appears to prolong life in mice, the *procyanidins* (condensed tannins) in red wine have proven to be the most potent polyphenol affecting the health and longevity of humans. Interestingly, red wines from southwest France and Sardinia have the highest procyanidin content, and these are also the areas with the greatest longevity in the French population. Grape seeds are the primary source of procyanidins, and the procyanidin content of red wines varies with the method of wine making and the type of grape used (greater exposure to grape pulp enhances wine's procyanidin content).[13]

IMBIBING BENEFITS HEART ATTACK SURVIVORS

Several studies have shown that for people who have been diagnosed with heart disease, light to moderate alcohol consumption lowers the risk of death from coronary artery disease by 20 to 50 percent.[14] Supporting the contention that a little wine benefits heart patients are the findings from a large Italian study published in the journal *Arteriosclerosis, Thrombosis, and Vascular Biology*. A cardiac catheterization was performed on more than two thousand male and female survivors of a heart attack or other cardiac event. For ten years following hospital discharge, the patients were monitored and their alcohol consumption habits recorded. Drinking in moderation, defined as at least 231 grams per week in men

---

MODERATE DRINKING AFTER STENT ANGIOPLASTY LOWERS RISK OF ARTERY NARROWING

Research published in the *British Medical Journal* has shown that heart disease patients who have undergone stenting (insertion of a small tube) of a coronary artery benefit from moderate drinking. The study involved 225 men who had undergone a procedure called balloon angioplasty to open up blocked coronary arteries. The risk is that the stent itself can cause inflammation, resulting in renewed narrowing of the stented artery—a rapid event that tends to occur within the first four months of the intervention. The men were divided into two groups based on alcohol consumption habits: greater than 50 grams of alcohol per week and less than 50 grams of alcohol per week. Of interest was that those who drank less alcohol had significantly lower HDL values as well as more extensive vessel disease. After six months, a second angiogram revealed that the men who drank more than 50 grams per week of alcohol (equating to at least four glasses of wine per week) were half as likely to require repeat angioplasty and significantly less likely to experience narrowing compared to men who drank little or no alcohol.

Source: F. Niroomand et al., "Influence of alcohol consumption on restenosis rate after percutaneous transluminal coronary angioplasty and stent implantation," *Heart* 90 (October 2004): 1189–1193.

(~2 drinks a day) and at least 154 grams per week in women (~1.5 drinks a day), was associated with significantly less atherosclerosis in the coronary arteries, an effect that translated into a lower risk of cardiac-related death over the ten-year period.[15]

The Determinants of Myocardial Infarction Onset Study examined the alcohol intake habits of 1,913 men and women within four days of surviving a heart attack. Death statistics of participants were then obtained for almost four years. Survival was lowest in those who were abstainers and highest in those consuming seven or more drinks per week. The scientists concluded that mild to moderate consumption of alcohol lessens risk of recurrent heart attacks and death in survivors of a cardiac event.[16]

Red wine cuts risk of a second heart attack in half

Modest wine drinking provides powerful protection for the hearts of cardiac patients against future heart attacks and lessens the chances of dying from heart disease. The Lyon study researchers examined the impact of moderate wine consumption on 437 middle-aged French men who were recent survivors of a heart attack. After a four-year follow-up, men who drank two or more glasses of red wine daily (each glass was about 4 fluid ounces) reduced their risk of a recurrent attack by more than 50 percent compared with nondrinkers.[17]

DAILY HEART DISEASE REVERSAL STRATEGY: RED WINE'S CONTRIBUTION

Strategy 1. Boost total antioxidant capacity and prevent LDL oxidation

Drinking a daily glass of red wine with your meal will contribute to raising your body's total antioxidant capacity (TAC), the way your body protects against damage to the inner lining of your blood vessel wall. You are now well aware of the power of plant polyphenols in raising your TAC and fighting off your disease. Repeated intake of plant antioxidants throughout the day is necessary for maintaining a high level of blood polyphenols—thus the Prevent a Second Heart Attack plan strategy to eat a variety of antioxidant-rich plant foods. Interestingly, the main sources of polyphenols in our diet are beverages, namely fruit juice, wine, tea, and coffee.[18] Laboratory studies indicate that drinking red wine has an immediate and potent TAC-boosting effect as reflected in blood levels determined by a scientific assay called the Oxygen Radical Absorbance Capacity (ORAC).[19]

Washing down your olive oil–drenched greens with a glass of pinot noir will triple your defenses against oxidative stress in your arteries. Remember, free radicals and oxidative stress play a crucial role in heart disease, because atherosclerosis is accelerated by the oxidation of LDL. Extra virgin olive oil is rich in the antioxidant tyrosol; greens are packed with potent flavonoids; and your glass of burgundy-hued wine is filled with powerful polyphenols, including resveratrol, which guards against LDL free radical attack. Pile them all together in the same meal and you have a synergistic action that fortifies your defenses against LDL oxidation with additional protective effects against atherosclerosis that are not as evident in any of the three foods alone.[20]

Go red and cut your LDL oxidation rate in half. Again, your choice of wine must be red and not white if you want to protect your LDL particles and heighten your defenses against oxidative stress. Scientists in Israel studied the effect of red versus white wine on LDL oxidation in seventeen healthy men. Half received 400 milliliters (~14 ounces) of red wine per day; the others were administered a similar amount of white wine for two weeks. Analysis of the subjects' blood yielded remarkable results, with the red wine cutting the subjects' LDL oxidation rate by more than 50 percent and substantially prolonging the lag time it took for the initiation of LDL oxidation. The white wine actually *increased* the LDL's propensity to undergo oxidation by 41 percent.[21]

Strategy 2. Raise your HDL cholesterol and rearrange cholesterol particle sizes

Consuming your daily red wine prescription will markedly raise your good HDL cholesterol level. Good HDL cholesterol is highly protective against atherosclerosis because it halts and reverses plaque formation.[22] Recall from Chapter 1 that low HDL (defined as less than 40 mg/dL) can greatly increase your risk for another heart attack and that individuals with really low HDL (<35 mg/dL) have *eight times* the risk of heart disease compared to those with high HDL (65 mg/dL or greater).[23]

Go red and boost your HDL level. Once again, the color of the wine really does matter. The same Israeli researchers who studied the effect of red wine on LDL oxidation gave seventeen healthy men 400 milliliters a day (about 13 fluid ounces) of either red or white wine for two weeks. Upon analysis of blood cholesterol level, only the red wine produced an impressive elevation in HDL cholesterol—26 percent after just two weeks![24]

Daily consistency of red wine drinking is an important factor in giving your HDL number a jolt upward. Previous research has shown that the increase in HDL gained from alcohol consumption is dose dependent, meaning the level rises in sync with the number of drinks per week.[25]

When it comes to HDL cholesterol, not only is more better, but you also want to have a high number of the larger, fuller version of HDL particles floating in your bloodstream. This is the type of HDL particle that is better at fighting off heart disease than the smaller version. Regular consumption of red wine can morph the shape of your HDL into the larger type, as was demonstrated by French researchers who analyzed the composition of HDL particles between drinkers and abstainers. Forty-six middle-aged French men participated in a study that provided a detailed analysis of HDL particle composition. The men were sorted into three groups depending on their typical daily alcohol intake: teetotalers, regular red wine drinkers, and heavy red wine drinkers. (Regular wine drinkers averaged 24 grams of alcohol daily—two 5-ounce glasses of wine; heavy drinkers averaged 47 grams of alcohol daily.) Results showed that the blood level of HDL level mirrored wine intake, with the heavier drinkers exhibiting the highest level. Not only were both groups of red wine drinkers' levels of HDL much higher than those of the abstainers, their HDL particles were markedly different. The drinkers' HDL particles were larger and filled with more cholesterol headed toward the liver for disposal. Also, the drinkers' HDL particles were enriched with the long-chain omega-3 fatty acid eicosapentaenoic acid, or EPA (the cardioprotective fish fat discussed in Chapter 9).[26]

Strategy 3. Help prevent blood clots by thinning your blood

Drinking a glass of red wine daily will render the platelets in your blood less sticky, lengthening the time it takes for them to congregate and form a deadly blood clot. Recall that a blood clot could block blood flow to the heart (the principal reason for a heart attack) or brain (stroke). Thus, wine has a similar effect to aspirin in its ability to thin the blood.

Go red and make your platelets less sticky. An Italian study compared the blood-thinning ability of red wine with that of white wine. Twenty healthy subjects were given 300 milliliters (10 ounces, or two glasses) a day of either red wine or white wine. At the end of the two-week trial period, each subject's blood was analyzed for platelet aggregation. Only the red wine decreased the blood's clotting ability, thanks to the two types of polyphenols found in high concentration in red wine, resveratrol and quercetin.[27]

Strategy 4. Decrease inflammation and improve artery health

Although mouse studies indicate that humans would have to consume 100 to 1,000 bottles of red wine a day to get the mouse equivalent of resveratrol for extending life, it appears that massive doses are not necessary for our arteries to derive the anti-inflammatory benefits. A new study of resveratrol's effects on mice has provided scientists with the first clues for exactly how this powerful red wine polyphenol can curtail inflammation. After examining the animal tissue, scientists from Scotland and Singapore found that mice that were administered resveratrol were unable to produce two molecules known to trigger inflammation.[28] Plus, resveratrol reduces your cells' production of inflammatory eicosanoids (the hormonelike substances formed from your body's metabolism of essential fatty acids) that are known to trigger atherosclerosis.[29]

Go red and make your artery wall less sticky. Drinking red wine will flood your blood vessels with potent polyphenols that decrease the number of adhesion molecules that surface from the endothelial cells.[30] This makes the endothelium less sticky so the artery's uptake of immune system cells—monocytes and T lymphocytes—will decline, which will help nip inflammation in the bud.

Go red and lower your CRP. Don't think you can substitute hard liquor such as gin for red wine and still garner the same heart health benefits. Although research has shown that all forms of alcoholic drinks, drunk in moderation, confer some cardioprotection, red wine is by far the superior choice. A study published in the journal *Atherosclerosis* pitched red wine against gin, measuring inflammatory biomarkers in the subjects' blood. Researchers gave forty healthy men either red wine or gin (30 grams of ethanol a day) for twenty-eight days. Both groups had a reduced level of a blood-clotting factor (suggesting that all forms of ethanol are effective at thinning the blood); however, only the red wine drinkers had dramatically reduced levels of inflammatory markers such as C-reactive protein (CRP) and endothelial cell adhesion molecules.[31]

Strategy 5. Regulate blood sugar to help prevent and treat type 2 diabetes

Drinking a little bit of alcohol in moderation can help lower your risk of developing type 2 diabetes. A meta-analysis, pooling the results from fifteen large-scale studies involving data drawn from nearly 370,000 individuals, revealed that compared with abstainers, moderate drinkers cut their risk of developing type 2 diabetes by 30 percent. *Moderate,* in this case, was defined as between 6 grams and 48 grams of alcohol a day, or about ½ to 3½ glasses of wine.[32]

One reason moderate alcohol consumption can have a favorable effect on your blood sugar has to do with insulin resistance—a condition in which the muscle, fat, and liver cells do not respond properly to the hormone insulin. Insulin resistance is part of metabolic syndrome, the constellation of metabolic disorders that accelerates atherosclerosis and is often a precursor to type 2 diabetes. Drinking lightly has been shown to increase your cells' sensitivity to insulin, which in turn helps thwart metabolic syndrome. When your cells become more sensitive to insulin, your body metabolizes sugar better, at least for twelve to twenty-four hours following alcohol ingestion. Hence the dictum to drink only a small amount of alcohol regularly—on a daily basis, and with food. A one-drink-a-day habit has been shown to lessen the likelihood of contracting metabolic syndrome by a phenomenal 40 percent.[33]

Strategy 6. Lower blood pressure and relax your arteries

Drinking your red wine prescription can increase the elasticity of your arteries, relaxing them and lowering the pulse rate, which results in a reduction in blood pressure. If you *have* been diagnosed with high blood pressure, you should know that data from more than fourteen thousand male doctors drawn from the Physicians Health Study supports the heart health benefits of light to moderate drinking in men with previously diagnosed high blood pressure. After a follow-up period of about 5.5 years, moderate drinking in men with high blood pressure was associated with a 44 percent reduced risk of dying from a heart attack compared to the doctors with high blood pressure who rarely or never drank.[34] But don't overdose on your liquid medicine, especially if you have diagnosed high blood pressure. There is evidence that alcohol intake in excess of two drinks per day can contribute to *raising* blood pressure, so make sure not to exceed the recommended daily limit of one to two drinks.[35]

Red wine (and especially the resveratrol and the quercetin in red wine) stimulates the production of nitric oxide, a compound known as a *vasodilator*, which relaxes blood vessels, reduces blood pressure, and improves vascular health. Nitric oxide is the heart-healthy substance (produced by endothelial cells) that is in short supply in cardiac patients—a major contributing factor to constricted and diseased vessels. If you don't produce enough nitric oxide, the result is stiff, inflexible, and unhealthy arteries. The solution? According to Italian scientists, regular (and of course moderate) wine consumption will enhance nitric oxide synthesis.[36]

A TOAST TO THE HEART HEALTH BENEFITS OF DRINKING WINE

Revere the purple grape! The data are clear: The simple and utterly enjoyable act of sipping a glass of fermented purple grape juice, with food, can help you prevent a second heart attack. A daily tipple of your favorite red, used to wash down your olive oil–infused Mediterranean-style meal, will add years to your life and life to your years. There is no greater pleasure than to sit down to a leisurely dinner of deliciously fresh whole food, artfully prepared, tempered with a flavorful glass of pinot noir, and shared with friends and family. In addition to helping you savor your food, red wine—a veritable cauldron of plant chemicals—can calm your nerves and lower your blood pressure, raise your HDL, rearrange your cholesterol particles and change their size, increase your insulin sensitivity, and lower arterial inflammation. If you can drink safely, then here's a toast that embodies my hope that you will live long and live well: To life, to life, *l'chaim!*

13

A Heart-Healthy Bonus: Dark Chocolate

There's more to life than chocolate, but not right now.

—Anonymous

 Eat 2 tablespoons of natural, unsweetened cocoa powder or one or two squares (up to 1 ounce) of dark chocolate (at least 70 percent cocoa) every day.

Companion foods R$_X$: several cups of green tea daily

Primary disease-fighting bioactive compounds:

- Cocoa polyphenol flavonoids, especially the flavonols: catechins, epicatechins, and procyanidins
- Green tea polyphenol flavonoids, especially the flavonols: epigallocatechin gallate (EGCG), epigallocatechin, epicatechin gallate, and epicatechin

The indigenous Kuna Indians, a population in Panama who mostly inhabit parts of the northern shore and the neighboring San Blas Archipelago, rarely develop high blood pressure and have a very low death rate from cardiovascular events compared with the Kuna Indians in urban Panama City. Why the difference in disease rates between the Kuna populations? It certainly isn't genetics. Scientists think the answer lies in the varying eating habits between the indigenous Kuna and their urban counterparts, specifically the fact that indigenous Kuna consume enormous amounts of superbly heart-healthy and flavonoid-rich cocoa—at least 5 cups every day.[1]

CHOCOLATE: FOOD OF THE GODS

Cacao is a small tropical tree whose seeds (beans) are used to make powdered cocoa and chocolate. Cultivation can be traced back thousands of years to the great Olmec settlements of Mesoamerica. Chocolate drinking vessels dating from approximately A.D. 450–500 have been found at the burial sites of the ancient Maya nobility of Mexico and Central America. Both the Maya and the Aztecs offered cacao as a gift to the gods, prompting Carl Linnaeus, the Swedish botanist and father of modern taxonomy, to name the cacao tree *Theobroma cacao,* literally "food of the gods." Cocoa as a beverage came to Europe in the sixteenth century, brought back by the discoverers of the New World, and in the nineteenth century it became a luxury item. In Britain in the early 1800s, cocoa was transformed from primarily a beverage (without sugar) into the solid chocolate confections (with added sugar and milk) that so many of us worship today.[2]

Cocoa and chocolate are two different things

After harvest, the beans from the cacao tree are fermented, dried, cleaned, and roasted, and then the nibs (the "meat" or center of the cocoa bean after the outer layer is removed) are ground into a thick, dark brown paste called *chocolate liquor.* Chocolate liquor consists of cocoa butter (fat) and cocoa solids (nonfat cocoa powder or finely ground cocoa beans). The fat in cocoa butter is mostly saturated, although one third is stearic acid, a saturated fat that has a neutral effect on blood cholesterol level.[3] Cocoa solids are the nonfat component of the liquor, whereas chocolate is a confection made of cocoa, cocoa butter, sugar, and sometimes milk, formed into a solid food product.

All cocoa solids are high in flavonoids—the polyphenol antioxidant component that makes chocolate "healthy." It's what happens next in processing that determines whether the final chocolate product retains the healthy flavonoids. Because flavonoids are bitter, manufacturers treat natural cocoa to remove much of the flavonoids, which will enhance flavor. *Dutching,* or alkalization of cocoa, for example, makes the chocolate taste milder and removes almost all of the flavonoids, so avoid purchasing Dutched chocolate products.[4] Although Dutch cocoa is intensely dark in color, it's not the depth of the color that should alert you to the health benefits of the product but the flavonoid content—which in Dutch chocolate has been severely depleted. (Note that quantification of the exact amount of flavonoids contained in commercial chocolate products is not available yet; however, it is likely that manufacturers will report those values in the not too distant future. Certain chocolate manufacturers, such as Mars and Barry Callebaut, have developed proprietary methods of processing cocoa that retains the flavonoid content.)

THE SWEET SCIENCE BEHIND DARK CHOCOLATE

Dark chocolate—with a high content of nonfat cocoa solids—is now the new guilt-free superfood! Isn't this the best nutrition news to come along in decades? The scientific evidence is stacking up linking daily consumption of deep, dark chocolate with phenomenal health benefits, especially on your heart and blood vessels. What's the magic ingredient in dark chocolate that confers the benefits? You guessed it—it's the flavonoids. And cocoa contains *lots* of flavonoids. In fact, dark chocolate has such a highly concentrated

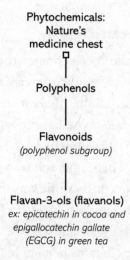

Phytochemicals:
Nature's
medicine chest

Polyphenols

Flavonoids
(polyphenol subgroup)

Flavan-3-ols (flavanols)
*ex: epicatechin in cocoa and
epigallocatechin gallate
(EGCG) in green tea*

Figure 13.1: Chocolate contains a large concentration of the flavonoid subgroup of polyphenols called flavan-3-ols, or flavanols.

amount of flavonoids that it beats out red wine. But what is perhaps more important than the concentration of flavonoids in dark chocolate is the type of flavonoid, which falls under the flavonol subclass (Figure 13.1), and contains the powerful subgroup called epicatechins.[5]

CHOCOLATE LOWERS ODDS OF DEATH FOLLOWING FIRST HEART ATTACK

In a recent study out of the Karolinska Institute in Stockholm, scientists found that people who eat chocolate (high in cocoa solids) have increased long-term survival rates following a heart attack. For eight years the researchers monitored nearly 1,200 middle-aged men and women who had been hospitalized for a recent heart attack. A survey of chocolate consumption over the year preceding the subjects' hospitalization revealed that compared with people who ate no chocolate, those who indulged up to once per week had a 44 percent reduced risk of dying from a subsequent heart attack, and those who ate it twice or more per week had a 66 percent reduced risk.

Source: Imre Jansky et al., "Chocolate consumption and mortality following a first acute myocardial infarction: The Stockholm Heart Epidemiology Program," *Journal of Internal Medicine* 266 (2009): 248–257.

Not all chocolate is created equally

Keep in mind that it's the cocoa component of chocolate that contains the flavonoids, so the higher percentage of cocoa, the more flavonoids. So, to sum it all up, it's best to choose dark chocolate that's high in cocoa—even if you have to sacrifice some of the taste (remember, more cocoa can sometimes mean less sugar, and more bitterness than sweet). The simple solution is to sample several different dark chocolate products until you find one that appeals to you. Watch out for the impostors such as white chocolate (not "real" chocolate because it is made solely from cocoa butter, sugar, and milk and therefore contains negligible flavonoids), hot chocolate mixes (low in flavonoids), and chocolate syrups and milk chocolate bars (also low in flavonoids).

Best chocolate choices. Of the six top-selling cocoa/chocolate products on the market today, it is important to know which contains the greatest antioxidant activity. Researchers at the Hershey Company analyzed the commercially available chocolate-containing products and found that the level of nonfat cocoa solids was the main factor in determining antioxidant activity. Predictably, the more nonfat cocoa solids in a product, the better. Natural cocoa powders (ground cocoa solids) had the highest level of flavonols followed by unsweetened baking chocolates, dark chocolates, and semisweet chocolate baking chips. Milk chocolate and chocolate syrup had the least amount.[6] Do your heart good—choose your chocolate wisely and opt for making your own sweet treats from cocoa powder.

Cocoa powder. So for the time being, because the cocoa solids contain the lion's share of the antioxidant polyphenols, and the cocoa butter is where most of the fat is, it is best (healthier) to consume chocolate concoctions made from unsweetened natural cocoa bak-

WASH DOWN YOUR DARK CHOCOLATE WITH GREEN TEA

Just like chocolate, tea is a form of plant food—and plants contain a plethora of phytochemicals that when stacked together will maximize the strength of your daily heart disease defense system. No doubt about it, a few daily cups of tea, and especially green tea, can provide cardiovascular protection via antioxidant and anti-inflammatory mechanisms.

There are three main varieties of tea—black, oolong, and green—and all are derived from the tea plant known as *Camellia sinensis*. (Countless herbal infusions are informally referred to as "tea," but these are unrelated to real tea produced from *Camellia sinensis*.) Teas are classified based on how the leaves are processed, with the leaves of green tea being the least processed of the three varieties. Green tea is dried but not fermented; hence it retains the greatest amount of polyphenols.

What exactly is in green tea that wards off heart disease? Researchers believe that the primary therapeutic component in green tea is another type of flavonoid, the catechin family of plant polyphenols, found in exceptionally high concentration. The most abundant of the green tea polyphenols is called epigallocatechin gallate, or EGCG for short. EGCG is believed to be the most active health-protective component in green tea. (Incidentally, green tea contains 40 percent more polyphenols than black tea.) According to researchers out of the University of Hong Kong, EGCG is a highly effective agent for lowering inflammation in the bloodstream as well as reducing oxidation of LDL, thereby protecting against plaque buildup. So let's get over the Boston Tea Party and borrow a nice tradition from the British—teatime in the afternoon—but let's make it green tea. Bottoms up for better heart health!

Sources: George L. Tipoe et al., "Green tea polyphenols as an anti-oxidant and anti-inflammatory agent for cardiovascular protection," *Cardiovascular & Haematological Disorders—Drug Targets* 7 (2007): 135–144; and Yuji Naito and Toshikazu et al., "Green tea and heart health," *Journal of Cardiovascular Pharmacology* 54, no. 2 (2009): doi: 10.1097/FJC.0b013e3181b6e7a1.

ing powder. Make sure the cocoa powder has been produced using the Broma process (and not Dutch processing with alkali). Look for the words *natural cocoa powder unsweetened* on the product label, such as for the Scharffen Berger brand of natural cocoa powder. And next time you have a craving for hot chocolate, don't let the rich dark chocolaty label on Hershey's Special Dark cocoa powder fool you. This cocoa powder is actually a blend of natural and Dutch-processed cocoas, and as a result, this product provides even fewer antioxidants than Hershey's regular brand of natural unsweetened cocoa.

Dark chocolate bars. That said, sometimes there's just nothing like a couple of small pieces of rich, creamy dark chocolate to end your meal. So here's a guide to sorting through the plethora of dark chocolate bars on the market to make sure that you are choosing a heart-healthy high-flavonoid chocolate product. Here are a few chocolate-choosing tips:

• Look at the ingredient list and make sure the first ingredient is cocoa or chocolate and not sugar.

• Look at the serving size. Your daily heart disease reversal prescription calls for no more than 20 grams (about two small squares) of solid dark chocolate. Keep in mind that chocolate is a treat and certainly not a low-calorie food. Most of the mammoth premium chocolate bars sold in the supermarket are 100 grams, with a serving described as three or four squares at about 40 grams (double what you should eat). Read the Nutrition Facts panel and zero in on the Calories, Total Fat, and Sugars numbers.

• Scan the ingredients label to ensure that the chocolate was not processed with alkali. For example, a 1.5-ounce bar of Godiva Chocoiste solid dark chocolate, which appears from the front label to be a heart-healthy dark chocolate bar, is actually processed with flavonoid-robbing alkali. A quick inspection of the ingredients list on the back label reveals the word *alkali*, which should prompt you to place this product back on the shelf.

Watch your sweet tooth. Make no mistake about it: Chocolate (as we know it) is in no way a diet food. It is often loaded with calories,

DECIPHERING THE CHOCOLATE FACTS ON THE WRAPPER

Your goal is to choose a bar that is highest in dry cocoa solids and lowest in fat and sugar (yet not too bitter for your palate). Let's make a comparison. Say you pick up a bar of Lindt Excellence 90% Cocoa. Check out the Nutrition Facts panel and you will see that one bar weighs 3½ ounces or 100 grams. Four squares (40 grams) is considered a serving and contains 210 calories, 20 grams of fat, and 3 grams of sugar. Glance at the ingredients list and you will see that the first ingredient is chocolate. Add the fat grams to the sugar grams and the total is 13 grams. Forty grams minus 23 grams equals 17 grams of mostly dry cocoa solids. Compare this to a Lindt Excellence 50% Cocoa bar. For the same serving size you get 200 calories, 15 grams of fat, and 18 grams of sugar. The first ingredient listed on this bar is sugar. Fifteen fat grams plus 18 sugar grams totals 33 grams. Forty grams minus 33 grams leaves you with just 7 grams of mostly dry cocoa solids in this product. *In general, the higher the percentage of cocoa advertised on the label, the better.* (Keep in mind that because you are only eating 2 squares, or up to 20 grams, you will be consuming just half the calories, fat, and sugar you calculated earlier.)

fat, and sugar, which is why if you choose to eat a chocolate confection, I suggest you make it no more than an ounce of at least 70 percent dark chocolate per day. The American Heart Association (AHA) recently included sugar on its blacklist of ingredients—joining the ranks of saturated fat, trans fat, dietary cholesterol, and sodium—foods that consumers need to limit for better heart health. The recommendation specifies "added sugars" as the primary offender—added sugars are sweeteners used by food processors to sweeten convenience foods such as soda, candy, fruit drinks, sweetened dairy products (sweetened yogurts, sweetened milk, and ice cream), cereals, and desserts.

The average American packs in about 22 teaspoons of added sugar daily. This translates into a daily addition of 355 empty calories. According to the AHA report, extra sugar intake can contribute to the development of obesity, insulin resistance, high blood pressure, high triglycerides, and type 2 diabetes—diseases and metabolic disorders that can accelerate atherosclerosis. The AHA recommends a maximum of 100 sugar calories for women (25 grams, or 6 teaspoons) and 150 calories for men (37 grams, or 9 teaspoons). Just how much added sugar is in your two squares of dark chocolate? There's approximately 13 grams of sugar (3 teaspoons) in a 1-ounce portion of a typical dark chocolate bar.[7] So your chocolate indulgence is well below the recommended daily intake, but you'll have to monitor your sugar intake elsewhere in your day. You may want to consider avoiding the sugar completely by whipping up your own chocolaty concoction using natural, unsweetened, dark cocoa powder and an artificial sweetener, such as my stunningly delicious Flourless Dark Chocolate Brownies with Walnuts (page 328). Or, if you simply want a quick chocolate fix (and don't feel like preparing anything), how about enjoying two small squares of Ghirardelli Chocolate Intense Dark Chocolate, Twilight Delight, 72% Cacao (110 calories, 5.5 grams of sugar, and the first ingredient is unsweetened chocolate!) and a cup of hot green tea?

DAILY HEART DISEASE REVERSAL STRATEGY: DARK CHOCOLATE'S CONTRIBUTION

Strategy 1. Boost total antioxidant capacity

Eating your daily sweet treat will make a significant contribution to the antioxidant potential of your diet, because dark chocolate has a higher antioxidant quality/quantity than most heavy hitters—red wine, black tea, and green tea.[8]

Swiss researchers performed an interesting study administering Nestlé Swiss (of course!) dark chocolate to twenty-two heart transplant patients. The patients were randomly divided into two groups and given 40 grams (~1.5 ounces) of either a dark chocolate bar with 70 percent cocoa or an equal amount of a flavonoid-free chocolate bar. (Individuals who have received a heart transplant are at risk for a condition called *transplantation-associated arteriosclerosis,* a rapidly progressing form of atherosclerosis that shortens transplant recipients' life span because of high oxidative stress and impaired nitric oxide production in the endothelial layer of their coronary arteries.) Two hours after the subjects ate the chocolates, their coronary arteries were examined for size and blood flow. The results? The blood concentration of epicatechin was greatly increased in the dark chocolate group, leading to an expansion of patients' coronary artery diameters and an elevation of their coronary blood flow—all good news for heart health. The ability of the platelets in the blood to stick to the inner artery wall of the dark chocolate eaters was also diminished—equally heart helpful, because it suggests that dark chocolate has potent anti-inflammatory *and* anti-clotting effects on the blood. (Note that the control group—eating the cocoa-free chocolate—did not exhibit any changes in their coronary arteries or blood flow.) The authors concluded that adding flavonoid-rich dark chocolate to the diet of heart disease patients is a simple and delicious lifestyle option that can effectively temper oxidative stress, the lethal plaque-building characteristic of these patients' coronary arteries that must be treated.[9]

Strategy 2. Lower your blood pressure

Eating flavonol-rich dark cocoa can also lower your blood pressure. A meta-analysis of five randomized, controlled clinical trials (the gold standard of research studies) has shown that regular consumption of flavonoid-rich cocoa reduces both systolic (top number) and diastolic (bottom number) blood pressure—at the same astonishing range as many blood-pressure-lowering medications.[10]

What if you have received a diagnosis of prehypertension, a condition in which your blood pressure is above normal but not quite high enough to classify you as having hypertension? Dark chocolate can help! A randomized, controlled, clinical trial of people with borderline high blood pressure showed that a small daily morsel of chocolate lowers blood pressure by a statistically significant amount, preventing progression to full-blown hypertension. The study divided forty-four prehypertensive men and women into two groups; one group received 6.3 grams of dark chocolate (about 0.25 ounce) daily and the other the same daily amount of a polyphenol-free white chocolate. After eighteen weeks, only the dark chocolate group showed a reduction in blood pressure numbers. What's more, the dark chocolate group showed a sustained increase in their blood level of the healthy blood vessel chemical nitric oxide.[11]

Why exactly does eating a small amount of dark chocolate affect your blood pressure? As noted in the Swiss study discussed earlier, when you ingest the main polyphenol in dark chocolate, epicatechin, it immediately activates the production of nitric oxide in the inner blood vessel wall; this in turn widens blood vessels and makes them more flexible, increasing blood flow and improving your blood pressure.[12]

Strategy 3. Make your dysfunctional endothelium more functional, especially if you're diabetic

Heart patients with diagnosed type 2 diabetes also receive exceptional benefit from dark chocolate. Drinking a nice big mug of hot chocolate is known to reverse endothelial dysfunction, and according to researchers out of Germany, it can make a significant difference even in people diagnosed with type 2 diabetes. Forty-one people taking medication for type 2 diabetes were randomly assigned to consume either a high dose (321 milligrams) of cocoa flavonols three times daily or a low dose (25 milligrams) three times daily for one month. The subjects' blood was then analyzed for polyphenol content. The high-dose flavonol-cocoa group had a notable increase in blood level of flavonols two hours after ingestion as well as a 30 percent increase in blood flow at the end of the study, which the authors attributed to a reversal of endothelial dysfunction in diabetics.[13]

Strategy 4. Lower inflammation in your arteries

As you learned, chronic low-level inflammation is a determinant in the onset and perpetuation of atherosclerosis. The simple act of indulging daily in a small amount of dark chocolate can help dampen the fire within your arteries. An Italian study has recently reported that a small square a day quells inflammation. And just a little (0.23 ounce) does the trick. More than two thousand healthy individuals underwent a blood test to determine the level of serum C-reactive protein (CRP), a protein in the blood that indicates inflammation in the arteries. The researchers related the levels of CRP with the subjects' usual intake of dark chocolate. A small amount of dark chocolate, eaten regularly, was associated with a 17 percent lower level of CRP.[14] And just like with red wine, a little is good but more is not better. In subjects consuming the highest amounts of chocolate (more than an ounce a day) the beneficial effect on inflammation all but disappeared—possibly because of the excess calorie intake. So aim for savoring up to 1 ounce (or two small squares) of dark chocolate a day, because eating more than that could possibly undo the healthful effects. Remember, a little goes a long way!

TIPS FOR GETTING IN YOUR DAILY DOSE OF DARK CHOCOLATE

• Try a nightly cup of steaming, decadent homemade hot chocolate. Put 2 heaping spoonfuls of dark chocolate cocoa powder (natural, unsweetened) into a mug, add a touch of sweetener (you might consider a sugar substitute), and mix together with soy milk and microwave. Top with fat-free whipped topping and you have a delicious, chocolaty, super-heart-healthy sweet treat.

• Remember, to satisfy your chocolate craving and fortify your heart disease defense strategy simultaneously, think real cocoa. Natural unsweetened cocoa powder has the highest concentration of flavonols compared to other chocolate products (followed by unsweetened baking chocolate), plus it is low in sugar, fat, and calories, so favor this chocolate choice over solid bars when possible. And don't forget that milk chocolate and chocolate syrup rank lowest on the antioxidant scale, so avoid choosing them for your heart-healthy chocolate splurge.[15]

• Look for dark chocolate products derived from single-origin countries or areas. Note that Madagascar and Java cacao beans have been shown to contain double the flavonols compared to beans from other areas.[16]

• If you prefer a small piece of chocolate, purchase one of the new high-flavonoid chocolate bars (not milk chocolate or Dutch processed)—at least 70 percent cocoa—and limit yourself to one to two small pieces a day. Be sure to check the ingredients list and choose a bar whose first ingredient is cocoa solids or chocolate (not sugar), such as Lindt Excellence 70% Cocoa Bar.

• Add a couple of tablespoons of dark cocoa powder to your banana and soy milk smoothie—a luscious addition to a heart-healthy drink.

CHOCOLATE: FOOD FOR THE HEART AND SOUL

Wonderful news for chocoholics! Intense, antioxidant-filled dark chocolate is no longer a forbidden food; we now know it contains a large amount of health-promoting bioactive compounds—flavonoids—more than the amount in many other plant foods (and yes, chocolate is a plant food and eating more plants and fewer animals is a wise nutrition philosophy). Consumption of the dark, flavonoid-rich type of chocolate can improve your blood vessel health by increasing your endothelium's production of that crucial blood vessel relaxation chemical nitric oxide, rendering your dysfunctional endothelium healthier and more functional.

Beware, however, because the devil is truly in the details when it comes to chocolate. Packaged with this delectable treat comes plenty of sugar and saturated fat and lots of calories that can pack on added pounds—negating the health effects. Many chocolates are made with milk or tropical oils (palm oil) and therefore contain an overload of LDL-raising saturated fat. The trick is to find the bar with the best ingredient profile and to eat just a small amount as part of your daily Prevent a Second Heart Attack plan. Better yet, go for the dark chocolate cocoa powder and add your own sweetener. One tablespoon of deep dark high-flavonoid cocoa powder, unlike chocolate, contains only 12 calories and zero grams of saturated fat and sugar.

So relish your daily dose of strong, divinely delicious chocolate, perhaps in combination with a soothing cup of green tea or a glass of your favorite red wine and give yourself a not-so-sinful indulgence—taking delight in the "food of the gods," enjoying life and halting heart disease the Prevent a Second Heart Attack Reversal Plan way.

Section 3

STAY ACTIVE: MOVEMENT = HEART HEALTH

Heart-Healthy Exercise: Walking

Walking is man's best medicine.

—Hippocrates, Greek physician (460–377 B.C.)

 Walk often and walk far.

Companion exercise R$_X$: supervised full-body strength training twice a week

Living a sedentary, couch-potato lifestyle is the American Way. But like so many of America's timeworn habits, it is a dangerous one— in fact, physical inactivity puts you at as great a risk for atherosclerosis as having diabetes does. Another gentle nudge into reality . . . after a heart attack, risk factors still continue to contribute to the progression of atherosclerosis in your blood vessels, and remaining sedentary is a *major risk factor*. I urge you to get those sneakers on every day because the good news is, the simple act of getting in daily exercise is the most powerful action you can take to tame your risk factors and decrease your odds of a second attack.[1] In people with heart disease, the benefits of starting and adhering to a regular program of walking—requiring only modest and certainly not a

Herculean effort—are no less than remarkable. Regular exercise builds up that extra network of blood vessels around blocked arteries called *collaterals* so that the heart muscles can get more blood flow. What's more, exercise can not only reduce progression but also promote *regression* of atherosclerosis, greatly reducing your odds of suffering a second attack, and can even extend your life. Hippocrates was truly the wisest of men when he stated more than two thousand years ago that "walking is man's best medicine."

EXERCISE BEATS STENTING FOR YEARLONG, EVENT-FREE SURVIVAL

German researchers performed an interesting study of 101 cardiac patients, pitting exercise training against insertion of a stent in the coronary artery to see which treatment benefited stable heart patients the most. The exercise group performed twenty minutes of stationary cycling a day in addition to one weekly sixty-minute group aerobics class; the stent group did not exercise. After one year, 88 percent of the exercisers were event-free (meaning these people did not have another heart attack or a dangerous episode of unstable angina) compared to 70 percent of the stented patients who were event-free. (The exercise therapy also cost significantly less than the medical stenting procedure!) The scientists concluded that exercise is a superior therapy for coronary patients *because it treats the entire diseased arterial tree,* whereas a stent targets only a small segment of the artery. They suggest that stenting (the current therapy of choice) without the addition of aggressive lifestyle therapy—including daily exercise, which slows the progression of atherosclerosis—should be viewed as a "suboptimal therapeutic strategy."

Source: Rainer Hambrecht et al., "Percutaneous coronary angioplasty compared with exercise training in patients with stable coronary artery disease: A randomized trial," *Circulation* 109 (2004): 1371–1378.

SURVIVAL OF THE FITTEST

It is well established that exercise training and an active lifestyle improve the prognosis of individuals with diagnosed coronary artery disease. A meta-analysis of data from thirty-two clinical trials involving nearly 8,500 heart patients showed that including exercise in the rehabilitation protocol for post–heart attack patients cut their death rate by a whopping 31 percent.[2]

The Corpus Christi Heart Project illustrated the phenomenal benefits of increasing your physical activity level after a first heart attack—proving that just a bit of exercise could improve your survival rate *and* reduce your odds of suffering another attack. More than four hundred survivors of a first heart attack were interviewed annually for seven years following their cardiac event. Patients who were physically active after their heart attack had *a 78 percent lower risk of having another heart attack and an 89 percent lower risk of death* compared to patients who remained sedentary.[3] No marathons required! A leisure activity such as walking is all that's necessary to achieve these miraculous benefits.

EXERCISE SAFETY

Worried that you could suffer a fatal heart attack during your exercise routine? Well, doctors disagree—exercise training is a medically recognized treatment that clearly improves prognosis for heart patients. There *is* a very small but real risk of having a cardiac event during exercise, but the statistics are encouraging—there are a reported two fatalities per 1.5 million cardiac patient hours of exercise.[4] Therefore, it is wise to talk with your personal physician about your risk for an exercise-related cardiac event and to find out whether exercise is right for you. If you get a green light following your post–heart attack stress test, your doctor may recommend that you participate in a supervised rehabilitation program as opposed to a home-based program. Also, if you have been sedentary for a long time, you *must* begin an exercise program gradually and cautiously, under your physician's supervision. (Your doctor should recommend that you undergo cardiac rehabilitation after your heart attack, especially if you have never exercised on a regular basis.) If all of this seems stressful or frightening, remember: It is actually riskier to forgo exercise entirely than to get in a bit of walking, so lace up your sneakers and enjoy some fresh air!

RED FLAG WARNINGS

• Consult with your personal physician for medical clearance before you begin any exercise program.

• Discuss with your physician whether it's safe for you to participate in a home-based exercise program; your doctor may want to refer you to an established, supervised cardiac rehab program.

• Restrict exercise intensity to moderate-resistance weight training and lower-level aerobic exercise.

• Do *not* exercise:

   • During the first week after a heart attack
   • If you have progressive and unstable angina
   • If exercise provokes atrial or ventricular arrhythmias
   • Within two weeks of having had uncomplicated coronary artery bypass surgery
   • If you have a postoperative infection

• Cease exercising and seek immediate medical attention if you experience chest pain, new or unusual abnormalities of cardiac rhythm, excessive breathlessness, or fatigue persisting more than a few hours.

Source: Paul D. Thompson, "Exercise prescription and proscription for patients with coronary artery disease," *Circulation* 112 (2005): 2354–2363.

WALKING: HOW MUCH, HOW OFTEN, AND HOW FAST

Walking is the most popular form of physical activity in the United States. In fact, not only is it popular, it is considered the best exercise prescription for fighting off heart disease. The medical consensus for post–heart attack patients is that walking should be the primary mode of exercise, done on a daily basis, working up to at least thirty minutes, and at a pace that is brisk yet permits you to talk comfortably.[5] Just how much should you be walking weekly? Studies show that if you burn at least 1,600 calories per week through exercise, you will halt the progression of atherosclerosis— and if you burn 2,200 calories per week, you can actually *reverse* the progression of atherosclerosis. These goals equate to walking fifteen and twenty miles a week, respectively.[6] The message? The intensity or speed of walking is not as important as the frequency and distance—walking a short distance very quickly burns as many calories as walking a long distance more comfortably.

More is better: Walk often, walk far

Researchers from the Division of Cardiology at the University of Vermont College of Medicine tested the somewhat archaic—yet still standard—protocols for cardiac rehabilitation, which typically recommend that patients burn a mere 700 to 800 calories per week in exercise. The researchers randomized seventy-four overweight subjects with coronary artery disease into two exercise groups. The control group exercised aerobically (walking, biking, or rowing) for twenty to forty minutes per session, three times a week, with the goal of burning 700 to 800 calories per week. The intervention group exercised five to seven days a week, walking for a longer duration (forty-five to sixty minutes), and at a lower intensity, with the aim of burning 3,000 to 3,500 calories per week. The basic motto for the intervention group was to "walk often, walk far." After five months, the high-calorie-burning exercise group, unsurprisingly, had double the weight loss and fat loss as well as greater loss of belly fat compared to the standard cardiac rehabilitation exercise group. What's more, the long walkers exhibited a greater reduction in insulin resistance and a greater increase in HDL cholesterol, as well as a decline in the prevalence of metabolic syndrome, from 59 percent of subjects assigned to the intervention group at the outset down to 31 percent at the end of the study. The long-duration walkers did not find this exercise prescription more difficult to accomplish (it was remarkably well accepted), nor did they experience an increased rate of overuse injuries compared to the control group. The authors concluded that this type of high-calorie-expenditure exercise should be the preferred protocol for almost 80 percent of cardiac rehab patients.[7] Your new mantra? *Walk often, walk far.*

STRENGTH TRAINING: GOOD FOR YOUR HEART, TOO

In addition to your daily walk, you may want to add in strength training—a regimen that can safely and effectively increase your muscle strength and endurance. This type of exercise benefits heart patients by favorably affecting heart function, modifying risk factors, enhancing psychological well-being, and improving quality of life. Stabilized cardiac patients are advised to partake in a resistance-training exercise program that meets the following criteria:

- Includes eight to ten different exercises targeting all the major muscle groups
- Uses weight that is light enough to permit one set of ten to fifteen repetitions of each exercise
- Involves doing a single set of each exercise as opposed to multiple sets
- Involves performing one set of each exercise at least twice weekly, on alternate days[8]

I recommend that you learn how to perform the strength training exercises under the careful supervision of a certified personal trainer or physical therapist versed in cardiac rehabilitation—don't just dive into a program on your own.

EXERCISE IS THE BEST MEDICINE FOR HEALING ARTERIES— BUT ONLY IF YOU STICK WITH IT!

Both types of exercise, aerobic exercise (such as walking) and strength training, either alone or in combination, safely improve blood vessel function in cardiac patients after a heart attack. However, after just one month of stopping exercise, the benefits on endothelial function all but vanish, according to a study reported in *Circulation: Journal of the American Heart Association.* Swiss researchers divided 209 recent heart attack survivors into one of four groups that for one month performed one of the following:

- Sixty minutes of cycling four times a week
- Resistance exercise four times a week
- Combined aerobic exercise two days a week and resistance exercise two days a week
- No exercise

LIFE IS GOOD IN COPENHAGEN: EXERCISE AND LIGHT DRINKING PROLONG LIFE

According to a recent "happiness" survey, the Danes are the happiest people in Europe. It comes as no surprise, then, that a large study out of Copenhagen found that moderate alcohol intake combined with regular physical activity is the best recipe for a long, happy, and low-stress life. Nearly twelve thousand Danish people were followed for approximately twenty years, providing data on level of physical activity, alcohol consumption habits, and other health statistics. The findings? Both being physically active and drinking at least one drink per week reduced the risk of a fatal heart attack by 50 percent compared to inactive nondrinkers.

Sources: The Economist "European Happiness Survey," April 19, 2007, http://www.economist.com/daily/chartgallery/displaystory.cfm?story_id=9030475; and Jane Østergaard Pedersen, "The combined influence of leisure-time physical activity and weekly alcohol intake on fatal ischemic heart disease and all-cause mortality," *European Heart Journal* 19 (2008): 204–212.

Researchers measured the endothelial function of the patients' brachial arteries both before and after the one-month trial. All three types of exercise caused a significant improvement in the functioning of the heart patients' arteries (an average increase in dilation from 4 to 10 percent), which the scientists noted could help slow the progression of atherosclerosis and fend off future heart attacks. Yet after a month of stopping the exercise regimen, the arterial benefits disappeared in all three exercise groups. The bottom line is, exercise is just like your medication: You will need to fill and take this prescription for life![9]

DAILY HEART DISEASE REVERSAL STRATEGY: EXERCISE'S CONTRIBUTION

Strategy 1. Improve your cholesterol

Putting on your sneaks *every day* and raising your heart rate will increase your level of "good" HDL cholesterol a considerable amount—but as I mentioned previously, the *frequency* of exercise is more important than the *intensity*. Recall from Chapter 1 the necessity of *both* lowering your LDL cholesterol and raising your HDL for maximum protection against future cardiac events. About half of the individuals who suffer a heart attack have a normal level of "bad" LDL cholesterol, which just goes to show you—LDL is only half of the heart disease equation![10] Equally important is your level of "good" HDL cholesterol—so remember, do what it takes to get your number *up to at least 40 mg/dL,* and higher is even better!

HDL plays several cardioprotective roles. Most important is its participation in the process called *reverse cholesterol transport*. HDL picks up excess cholesterol (the kind that contributes to plaque buildup) from inside the arterial wall and escorts it back to the liver for excretion. HDL also functions as an antioxidant: blocking LDL oxidation, protecting against excess LDL entry into the blood vessel wall, inhibiting adhesion molecule expression, and actively removing LDL from inside the endothelium. All of these factors make *HDL one of your strongest allies in heart attack prevention because of its ability to reverse the propensity of vulnerable plaque to rupture.*[11]

Exercise morphs LDL size from small to large. Recall that the small, dense LDL cholesterol particles, which doctors refer to as *pattern B,* are the most dangerous type. For maximum cardioprotection, it is best to get the total number of LDL particles down as low as you can *and* to change their size from pattern B to *pattern A* (large, fat, and fluffy). Exercise has been clinically proven to achieve this feat.[12] Making a concerted effort to take your daily exercise prescription is the safest and most effective strategy for "fluffifying" your bad LDL, especially if you follow the mantra "Walk often, walk far."

Strategy 2. Soothe inflammation and improve endothelial function

As you know, heart disease is partly caused by reactive oxygen, including free radicals, and the condition known as oxidative stress. Oxidative stress damages the delicate cells of your arteries, triggering inflammation and eventually leading to complications of atherosclerosis (heart attack). Chronic inflammation and endothelial dysfunction go hand-in-hand in promoting plaque vulnerability. Taking steps to dampen inflammation and reverse dysfunction in your arteries is therefore vital for the treatment and reversal of heart disease. Exercise is the best medicine for treating both conditions.

Recall that oxidative stress occurs when we have either an *overproduction* of destructive free radical molecules or an *impairment* of our natural antioxidant defense system. Thus, oxidative stress results when there is an imbalance between harmful pro-oxidant substances and helpful antioxidants. But how do you lower the amount of pro-oxidant substances within your body and boost your antioxidant army? Simple: You up your antioxidant ante. To accomplish this, you can draw from two pots: your own cells, which produce antioxidants naturally, and the food you eat.

EXERCISE COOLS THE FLAMES OF ARTERIAL INFLAMMATION

Inflammation is deeply involved in creating and destabilizing the plaque that has invaded your heart's blood vessel walls. Stop this inflammation in its tracks, and you take a major step in fighting your disease. Mounting scientific evidence shows that regular exercise acts like cortisone for the arteries—putting out the arterial flames.

Several types of blood tests are used to measure markers of inflammation in your arteries: high-sensitive (sometimes called *cardio* or *ultraquantitative*) C-reactive protein (hs-CRP) is one such marker. A high level of hs-CRP ($\geq$3 mg/L) indicates excessive arterial inflammation. Israeli scientists put twenty-eight patients with diagnosed heart disease into a twelve-week cardiac rehabilitation exercise program (mixed aerobic exercises: cycling, treadmill, and rowing, three times a week). Before the program, 72 percent of participants had a blood hs-CRP level greater than 3 mg/L, classifying them as "high risk." At the end of the study, there was a 46 percent reduction in the number of subjects in the high-risk category, supporting the researchers' conclusion that aerobic exercise training is an effective means to lower inflammation and improve risk in heart patients.

Source: Ehud Goldhammer et al., "Exercise training modulates cytokines activity in coronary heart disease patients," *International Journal of Cardiology* 100 (2005): 93–99.

Low antioxidant production is characteristic of heart patients. People with heart disease make very little of their own antioxidants. The two key "homemade" antioxidant enzymes—that is to say, chemicals that help produce antioxidants—are scientifically called *glutathione peroxidase* and *superoxide dismutase*. Research shows that patients undergoing bypass surgery often have a remarkably weak antioxidant capacity of glutathione, meaning their arteries don't have the raw material needed to create antioxidants.[13] What does this mean for you if you are living with heart disease? You need to do whatever it takes to heighten both your internal antioxidant production *and* your daily intake of antioxidant-rich foods to treat your disease. Getting in your daily exercise is an especially powerful method for intensifying your homemade endothelial cells' production of the free radical–disarming antioxidant enzymes (glutathione peroxidase and superoxide dismutase) that combine to toughen up your fight against inflammation and oxidative stress in your coronary arteries.[14]

Exercise boosts antioxidant production and reverses a dysfunctional endothelium. Exercise really does change your blood vessel physiology. Specifically, exercise eases your arteries' endothelial dysfunction by increasing your cells' production of nitric oxide. Recall that nitric oxide is the potent blood vessel relaxation chemical—much like the nitroglycerin tablets you may put under your tongue to ease the pain of angina. When the endothelial cells of your arteries become damaged, nitric oxide becomes limited. This shortage of nitric oxide leads to a series of problems—an increase in free radicals, increased adhesion molecule formation and sticking of white blood cells, increased permeability of the inner blood vessel layer, increased tendency for the blood to clot, and an impaired ability of blood vessels to dilate—all of which exacerbate plaque formation. According to two German physicians, *nitric oxide is the most important natural anti-atherosclerotic defense within your blood vessels.*[15] Regular exercise increases blood flow within the arteries, which stimulates your endothelial cells' production of nitric oxide. Therefore, regular exercise is your best medicine for restoring the synthesis of this lifesaving molecule.[16]

Strategy 3. Prevent or reverse metabolic syndrome

The simple act of taking a daily walk in the park will improve your cells' sensitivity to insulin. Metabolic syndrome, also known as *insulin resistance syndrome,* is often a precursor to developing type 2 diabetes as well as a major contributor to plaque buildup in your arteries. According to a scientific statement from the American Heart Association on cardiac rehabilitation, exercise, and the prevention of secondary cardiac events, aerobic exercise can favorably modify all of the components of metabolic syndrome. The scientific paper clearly states that exercise training should be *first-line therapy* in cardiac patients to combat both metabolic syndrome and heart disease.[17]

Strategy 4. Lower blood pressure

Getting in your daily exercise prescription is highly effective medicine for controlling blood pressure because of the link between exercise and the boost in nitric oxide production (when nitric oxide relaxes and dilates the blood vessels, the effect is to lower blood pressure). Physical activity increases blood flow, resulting in a healthy dose of *shear stress,* a healthy stressor that triggers dilation of the vessels and the increase in nitric oxide production. A Brazilian study has shown just how effective exercise is for treating blood pressure. Researchers found that six months of moderate-intensity exercise training (stationary bicycling for sixty minutes, three days a week) was enough to increase nitric oxide level by an incredible 60 percent. Eleven sedentary, postmenopausal women with diagnosed high blood pressure were recruited for the study. At the end of the six-month period, systolic blood pressure (top number) dropped 12 percent and diastolic (bottom number) 10 percent. What's more, the women's total cholesterol numbers also fell by an average of 20 percent.[18]

Strategy 5. Lose weight

Make no mistake about it, losing excess body fat is one of your most powerful weapons in your fight against heart disease. Being overweight affects your arteries, making them more prone to plaque formation. Attaining a healthy body weight—and losing body fat, especially artery-clogging belly fat—will greatly contribute to the reversal of your disease process. Becoming overweight is the result of routinely consuming too many calories combined with burning too few (physical inactivity). To lose weight in a healthful manner and in a way that doesn't tax your heart, aim for a gradual weight loss of no more than one to two pounds per week by eating nutritious calorie-controlled meals combined with daily calorie-burning exercise. Ideally, it is best to achieve a body mass index (BMI)—an indicator of body fat based on height and weight—of less than 25, according to government recommendations.[19] (Refer to the National Heart, Lung, and Blood Institute's Web site, *http://www.nhlbisupport.com/bmi/,* for an online BMI calculator, or simply search for a BMI calculator in any search engine.)

A healthy rate of weight loss is attained when you create a calorie deficit—a situation in which you consistently expend more calories than you consume. Creating a calorie deficit of 3,500 calories in a week equates to a loss of 1 pound of body fat. By partaking in the high-calorie-expenditure walking exercise prescription promoted in the Prevent a Second Heart Attack plan, you will find it easier to accomplish your weight-loss goals.

TIPS FOR GETTING IN YOUR DAILY DOSE OF EXERCISE

• Make walking a priority in your life, just like taking your medication. If you cast a positive light on exercise and acknowledge that it is the best medicine for promoting healing, for improving your joie de vivre, and especially for releasing harmful plaque-promoting stress, then you will be more likely to embrace this lifetime prescription.

• Start slow, maybe just a walk around the block, and build up over time to your set distance.

• Set a target, choose a set distance, and plan to walk that distance and back—every day.

• Wear the right clothes and the right shoes. Remember to hydrate before and after your walk, and remember to protect yourself against the elements.

• Walk with a buddy or your dog if you prefer company; this may make walking more enjoyable for you.

• Purchase a portable music player and listen to your favorite tunes while you walk off your stress.

• Walk indoors on a treadmill—place it in front of the television and walk during your favorite show.

• Hire a personal trainer—if you pay for strength training you will more likely go for your appointment. Contact a personal training studio near you.

TAKE THE WALK OF LIFE

Imagine a medication that could raise your HDL cholesterol, lower your blood pressure, prevent diabetes, increase your blood vessels' production of nitric oxide, give you more energy, enable you to lose body fat, and make you feel happy to be alive. That medicine exists, it's free, and it's called walking! Adding physical activity to one's daily routine has been proven to lengthen the life span and retard the appearance of age-related disabilities. Without question, getting an adequate amount of daily exercise protects against heart disease and helps balance calorie expenditure and intake, making it much easier to maintain weight control. At least thirty minutes a day of increased physical activity works its magic as an anti-inflammatory salve. Regular activity is especially valuable for managing blood sugar level, as it increases the muscles' sensitivity to insulin.

The scientific evidence is rock solid: More than twenty years of data has documented that exercise combined with diet can mitigate progression of atherosclerosis and reverse existing disease.[20] Know that these multiple lifestyle habits (eating the foods described in these pages and getting in your daily exercise), when practiced together with your prescription medication regimen, will provide you with the most powerful plan of action known to modern medicine to fight, halt, and reverse heart disease, making you, the "vulnerable patient," clearly much less vulnerable, if not invincible.

A Few Closing Words from Dr. Janet

You have heart disease, and you know it's a lifelong condition. The good news is that you can control it—and also live a long and rewarding life. You and you alone are the architect of your health, and you have the tools to build as happy and long a life as you'd like. There is so much you can do to reverse plaque buildup in your coronary arteries, stabilize vulnerable plaque, and target the three areas of vulnerability that ultimately will prevent that second attack.

As I'm sure you know by now, my Prevent a Second Heart Attack plan is not a diet of deprivation, but rather of delicious food combined with an active lifestyle that will help you be happier and healthier than ever before. The Prevent a Second Heart Attack plan is a Mediterranean-style eating strategy that incorporates the traditional healthy living habits of the people of Crete in the early 1960s, back when their cuisine was natural and fresh—like the crystal clear Aegean Sea that was home to the harmonious blend of fish and fauna the Cretans ate with such passion. What a contradiction to the rich, artery-clogging animal foods that we Americans are still glutting on today!

The dietary theme set out in these pages is that good-for-you food can also be *good* food. The foods described in the pages of the Prevent a Second Heart Attack plan—vegetables, fruits, legumes, whole grains, nuts, seeds, olive oil, fish, and a glass or two of red wine with dinner—are fresh, unprocessed, unrefined, and low in saturated fat, trans fats, and dietary cholesterol. My plan is not a diet per se but a synergy of complementary *whole foods that when eaten in combination reverse heart disease.* No one food, pill, or dietary supplement alone can stop plaque buildup and mimic the extraordinary health benefits obtained from this back-to-basics plan of healthy eating and physical activity.

Take this book to heart and it will be an invaluable tool for helping you, a heart attack survivor, to live a lifestyle designed and tested to guard against that second and often fatal heart attack. Even more, it will allow you to continue to enjoy food and the good things in life. I encourage you to "eat like you're in Crete," and in so doing you will be living a protective lifestyle designed to target the three vulnerable areas that contribute to your risk of getting another attack: (1) stabilizing vulnerable plaque and reducing inflammation, (2) stabilizing the electrical conductivity of your heart muscle, and (3) changing the composition of your blood—all while adding vibrant years to your life. Again, you have the power to change your health by the lifestyle choices you make today.

Best wishes for a long and happy life.

A toast to your health!

—*Dr. Janet Brill*

Part III

The Prevent a Second Heart Attack Plan in Action

Section 1

14-DAY MEAL PLAN

15

Meal Plan—14 Days of Eating Your Way Back to Health

Nothing would be more tiresome than eating and drinking if God had not made them a pleasure as well as a necessity.

—François-Marie Arouet de Voltaire, French Enlightenment writer and philosopher (1694–1778)

PUTTING IT ALL TOGETHER

So what does a day of eating look like when you live the Prevent a Second Heart Attack way? Table 1 shows you just how to get your eight foods in, followed by two sample weeks of meal plans. Try to eat at least the suggested variety of fresh fruit and vegetables—using extra virgin olive oil liberally to flavor your food. Adjust your portion sizes to control your weight, and remember to get your daily exercise in. The checklist in the Appendix is a helpful tool—it will aid you in balancing out your Prevent a Second Heart Attack day, your way. Bon appétit!

Table 1.

SAMPLE ONE-DAY MENU INCORPORATING THE EIGHT
PREVENT A SECOND HEART ATTACK FOODS

Meal	Food	Food Checklist
Breakfast	Oatmeal	✓ Whole grain
	Ground flaxseeds	✓ Flaxseeds (omega-3 ALA)
	Soy milk	✓ Legume
	Mixed berries	✓ Fresh fruit
Snack	Walnuts and dried figs	✓ Walnuts (omega-3 ALA)
		✓ Figs
Lunch	Greek salad:	✓ Vegetables, herbs (onions, garlic)
	Tomatoes, onions, cucumber, peppers, garlic, olives, a very small amount of low-fat feta cheese, dressed with olive oil, vinegar, and fresh lemon juice	✓ Olives ✓ EVOO ✓ Fresh fruit
	Whole-grain pita sandwich stuffed with:	✓ Whole grain
	Hummus	✓ Legume, garlic, EVOO
	Assorted vegetables	✓ Vegetables
Snack	Apple and cantaloupe slices	✓ Fresh fruit
Dinner	Glass of red wine	✓ Red wine with meal
	Salmon seasoned with olive oil, garlic, dill, capers, and lemon	✓ Fatty fish (omega-3 EPA/DHA), EVOO, garlic, herbs, and fruit
	Lentils served over brown rice	✓ Legume
	Spinach sautéed with garlic and olive oil	✓ Whole grain
		✓ Vegetable (dark leafy green), garlic, EVOO
	2 squares dark chocolate for dessert	✓ Dark chocolate

ALA = alpha-linolenic acid; EVOO = extra virgin olive oil; EPA = eicosapentaenoic acid; DHA = docosahexaenoic acid

Sample Week One: PREVENT A SECOND HEART ATTACK MEAL/EXERCISE SCHEDULE

	Monday	Tuesday	Wednesday	Thursday	Friday	Saturday	Sunday
	Walk at least 30 minutes/ strength train	Walk at least 30 minutes/ strength train	Walk at least 30 minutes	Walk at least 30 minutes/ strength train	Walk at least 30 minutes	Walk at least 30 minutes	Walk at least 30 minutes
Breakfast	Oatmeal raisin muffins♥ Fresh blueberries	**Breakfast** *(on the road at a chain establishment such as Au Bon Pain or Starbucks):* Oatmeal with raisins, almonds, brown sugar and fat-free milk/ flaxseeds Berries	**Breakfast** Steel-cut oatmeal♥ Soy milk Flaxseeds Dried cranberries Fresh mango with lime	**Breakfast** Spinach egg-white omelet Soy sausages 100% whole-wheat toast Grapefruit segments	**Breakfast** Cold oatmeal♥ Soy milk Flaxseeds Dried cranberries	**Breakfast** Steel-cut oatmeal Soy milk Flaxseeds Dried cranberries Melon	**Breakfast** Oatmeal-walnut pancakes Fresh raspberries
Snack	Walnuts with fat-free Greek yogurt, dried figs, Splenda if desired	**Snack** Walnuts with fat-free Greek yogurt, dried figs, Splenda if desired	**Snack** Walnuts with fat-free Greek yogurt, dried figs, Splenda if desired	**Snack** Walnuts with fat-free Greek yogurt, dried figs, Splenda if desired	**Snack** Walnuts with fat-free Greek yogurt, dried figs, Splenda if desired	**Snack** Walnuts with fat-free Greek yogurt, dried figs, Splenda if desired	**Snack** Starbucks soy latté Dried figs
Lunch	Linguine with Fresh Vegetables♥ Whole-wheat pita	**Lunch** *(brown bag)* Almond nut butter and banana sandwich on 100% whole-wheat bread Bag of mini carrots	**Lunch** Fresh veggie pita pocket sandwich♥	**Lunch** Roasted tomato soup♥ Soy deli turkey and veggie sandwich on 100% whole-wheat bread Baked potato chips	**Lunch** Salsa with light tortilla chips Vegetarian Mexican bean wrap♥	**Lunch** At the Japanese restaurant: Edamame Miso soup Assorted sashimi Brown rice	**Lunch** Turkey and bean chili♥

Monday	Tuesday	Wednesday	Thursday	Friday	Saturday	Sunday
Snack Apple	**Snack** Starbucks soy latté Orange	**Snack** Apple	**Snack** Cannellini bean dip with pita chips♥ Apple	**Snack** Soy yogurt Fresh blackberries	**Snack** Veggies/hummus♥	**Snack** Nectarine
Dinner* Apple-Carrot salad♥ Salmon with braised lentils♥ Dinner roll with EVOO	**Dinner*** Yellowtail en papillote♥ Spinach with pine nuts and raisins♥ Wild rice salad♥	**Dinner*** Steamed halibut with vegetables in parchment♥ Roasted beets with lemon vinaigrette♥ Curried whole-wheat couscous♥	**Dinner*** Arugula salad with figs and walnuts♥ Shrimp with artichoke-garlic sauce♥ Barley mushroom pilaf♥	**Dinner*** Green pea and lima bean soup♥ Grilled swordfish♥ Roasted Brussels sprouts♥ Quinoa with walnuts♥ Whole-grain bread dipped in EVOO	**Dinner*** Basil pesto crostini♥ Mixed greens with shallot vinaigrette♥ Whole-grain pasta with roasted eggplant, olives, and tomatoes♥	**Dinner*** Mixed greens with parsley-chive dressing♥ Ratatouille with whole-grain pasta♥ Brown rice
Green tea Dark chocolate	Green tea Dark chocolate	Green tea Dark chocolate	Hot chocolate	Green tea Dark chocolate	Green tea Dark chocolate	Green tea Chocolate brownies♥

♥ Heart-healthy recipe included   * Optional glass or two of red wine with dinner EVOO = extra virgin olive oil

Sample Week Two: PREVENT A SECOND HEART ATTACK MEAL/EXERCISE SCHEDULE

	Monday	Tuesday	Wednesday	Thursday	Friday	Saturday	Sunday
	Walk at least 30 minutes	Walk at least 30 minutes/ strength train	Walk at least 30 minutes	Walk at least 30 minutes/ strength train	Walk at least 30 minutes	Walk at least 30 minutes	Walk at least 30 minutes
Breakfast	Cold oatmeal♥ Soy milk Flaxseeds Dried cranberries Kiwi slices	*(at the diner)* Oatmeal with cinnamon, raisins, and slivered almonds/flaxseeds Cantaloupe	Steel-cut oatmeal♥ Soy milk Flaxseeds Dried cranberries Fresh strawberries	Cold oatmeal♥ Soy milk Flaxseeds Dried cranberries Fresh papaya with lime	Egg-white omelet with spinach 100% whole-wheat toast Grapefruit sections	Steel-cut oatmeal♥ Soy milk Flaxseeds Dried cranberries Fresh orange sections	Oatmeal-walnut pancakes♥ Fresh blueberries
Snack	Walnuts with fat-free Greek yogurt, dried figs, Splenda if desired	Walnuts with fat-free Greek yogurt, dried figs, Splenda if desired	Walnuts with fat-free Greek yogurt, dried figs, Splenda if desired	Walnuts with fat-free Greek yogurt, dried figs, Splenda if desired	Walnuts with fat-free Greek yogurt, dried figs, Splenda if desired	Walnuts with fat-free Greek yogurt, dried figs, Splenda if desired	Walnuts with fat-free Greek yogurt, dried figs, Splenda if desired
Lunch	Spinach salad♥ Lentil soup♥	Whole-wheat pizza with arugula, eggplant, and caramelized onions♥	Portobello pizzas♥ Roasted red pepper strips♥ Whole-grain pita	Roasted red pepper hummus♥ and vegetables on whole-grain wrap	Tuna and cannellini bean salad♥ Whole-grain pita	At the Chinese restaurant: Steamed tofu stir-fry with veggies Brown rice Green tea/2 fortune cookies	Red lentil curry♥

Snack	Dinner*	Beverage
Pear Soy nuts	**Apple carrot salad**♥ Pan-seared salmon Roasted cauliflower♥ Oven-roasted potatoes	Green tea Dark chocolate
Apple Soy crisps	Spinach salad with orange slices and olive oil vinaigrette Steamed red snapper with black bean sauce♥ Pea pods with almonds♥ Brown rice	Hot chocolate♥
Apple	**Arugula salad**♥ Grilled tuna Romesco♥ Chickpeas with roasted peppers♥	Green tea Dark chocolate
Baba ghanoush♥ on whole-wheat pita chips♥	Spinach salad with apples, walnuts, and dried cranberries♥ Mussels marinara♥ Side of whole-grain pasta Kale with white beans♥	Green tea Chocolate brownies♥
Baby carrots Peach	Greek Salad♥ Branzino with broccoli rabe♥ Barley mushroom pilaf♥	Green tea Dark chocolate
Apple	Spinach salad with orange slices and olive oil vinaigrette Whole-grain bread dipped in EVOO Herbed red beans and brown rice♥ Braised red cabbage with olives♥	Green tea Dark chocolate
Raw veggies with hummus dip♥	At the steakhouse: Salad bar: spinach, assorted veggies, chickpeas, and olive oil vinaigrette Grilled salmon Baked sweet potato Steamed broccoli	Green tea Dark chocolate

♥ Heart-healthy recipe included   * Optional glass or two of red wine with dinner   EVOO = extra virgin olive oil

Section 2

RECIPES

16

Prevent a Second Heart Attack Recipes

PREVENT A SECOND HEART ATTACK RECIPE TIPS FOR SUCCESS

Cooking with fresh seafood, vegetables, fruits, and grains forms the foundation of the two-week meal plan. For the best flavor and results when cooking our recipes, we recommend the following:

• Fresh fish fillets, mussels, and shrimp. If frozen fish or shrimp is used, thaw it completely before proceeding with the recipe. When cooking the fish, remember that most fish fillets need to cook for about 10 minutes per inch of thickness to be fully cooked.

• Kosher salt instead of table salt for a clean flavor and salt that readily dissolves. Per teaspoon, kosher salt contains about half the amount of sodium in table salt because of the larger size of the salt crystals. You can always use less salt than specified in the recipes, but the amount of kosher salt is a guideline for how to get the best flavor with the minimal amount of sodium.

- Reduced-sodium chicken or vegetable broth
- Fresh chopped herbs unless otherwise specified
- Freshly squeezed lemon and orange juice
- Fresh medium-sized garlic cloves, peeled and then minced or chopped
- Freshly ground black pepper
- White wine you would drink, such as Chardonnay, not a cooking wine
- Extra virgin olive oil in all recipes
- Canned beans, drained and rinsed
- And finally, enjoy your time in the kitchen, using fresh, high-quality ingredients to cook delicious, freshly prepared meals and snacks.

DR. JANET'S STEEL-CUT OATS
WITH FRESH FRUIT AND WALNUTS

SERVES 4

This oatmeal begs for improvisation. Be creative in substituting other fruits such as banana, chopped pear, or even dried blueberries or raisins for the apple.

> 1 cup steel-cut oats
> ½ teaspoon ground cinnamon
> ½ cup plain soy milk
> ¼ cup ground flaxseeds
> 1 large apple, peeled, cored and chopped
> ¼ cup chopped walnuts, toasted if desired

In a large saucepan bring 4 cups water to a boil. Stir in the oats and cinnamon. Reduce the heat and cook for 25 minutes. Stir in the soy milk and flaxseeds and cook for 5 more minutes. Serve topped with the chopped apple and walnuts.

NUTRITION PER 1-CUP SERVING

CAL	FAT*	SAT FAT	CHOLEST	SODIUM	CARB	DIET FIBER	SUGARS	PROTEIN
290	11 g	1 g	0 mg	26 mg	39 g	9 g	6 g	11 g

*FAT: 0 g EPA; 0 g DHA; 2 g ALA

From the kitchen of Dr. Janet

IN THE NUTRITION INFORMATION FOLLOWING EACH RECIPE

CAL=calories; SAT FAT=Saturated Fat; CARB=Carbohydrate;
CHOLEST=Cholesterol; DIET FIBER=Dietary Fiber

CHEF KEITH BLAUSCHILD'S OATMEAL RAISIN MUFFINS

SERVES 6

Mix the dry ingredients the night before, then finish the batter in the morning to start your day with a freshly baked muffin.

Nonstick cooking spray
¼ cup raisins
½ cup whole-wheat flour
¼ cup all-purpose flour
¼ cup quick-cooking rolled oats
¼ cup packed light brown sugar
½ teaspoon baking powder
¼ teaspoon ground cinnamon
½ cup unsweetened applesauce
¼ cup fat-free milk
2 large egg whites
1 tablespoon flaxseed oil

Preheat the oven to 375°F. Lightly coat six 2½-inch muffin cups with nonstick cooking spray or line with paper baking cups and coat the insides of the cups with nonstick cooking spray; set aside. Place the raisins and 2 tablespoons water in a small microwave-safe bowl. Microwave on high power for 25 seconds. Let sit for 2 minutes to plump the raisins.

In a medium bowl, stir together the flours, oats, brown sugar, baking powder, and cinnamon. Make a well in the center of the flour mixture and set aside. In a small bowl, combine the applesauce, milk, egg whites, flaxseed oil, and raisins. Add to the flour mixture; stir just until incorporated. Don't overmix. Spoon the batter into the prepared muffin cups, filling each about three-fourths full. Bake for 20 to 22 minutes, or until the muffins are lightly browned and firm in the middle. Cool in the pan on a wire rack for 5 minutes. Remove from the pan and serve warm.

NUTRITION PER 1 MUFFIN SERVING

CAL	FAT*	SAT FAT	CHOLEST	SODIUM	CARB	DIET FIBER	SUGARS	PROTEIN
157	3 g	<1 g	<1 mg	69 mg	30 g	2 g	13 g	4 g

*FAT: 0 g EPA; 0 g DHA; 1 g ALA

From the kitchen of
Parkland Chef Catering
2151 Riverside Drive
Coral Springs, Florida

DR. JANET'S OATMEAL, WALNUT, AND FLAXSEED PANCAKES

SERVES 6

Serve warm, sprinkled with fresh berries, a touch of powdered sugar, and fat-free whipped topping for a real Sunday morning treat (for you and your arteries!).

  1 cup 100% whole-wheat flour
  ½ cup old-fashioned oat flakes, ground
  ¼ cup ground flaxseeds
  ¼ cup finely chopped walnuts
  1½ teaspoons baking powder
  ½ teaspoon baking soda
  ½ teaspoon kosher salt
  1¼ cups light soy milk
  ¼ cup pure maple syrup
  1 large egg white
  Nonstick cooking spray
  Powdered sugar, optional
  Fat-free whipped topping
  Fresh berries

In a medium bowl, combine the flour, oat flakes, flaxseeds, walnuts, baking powder, baking soda, and salt. In another medium bowl, combine the soy milk, syrup, and egg white. Add the soy milk mixture to the dry ingredients and whisk just until incorporated. Coat a large frying pan with nonstick cooking spray. Heat the pan over medium heat. Spoon in four circular pancakes, about ¼ cup each. Cook until the batter bubbles, then flip with a spatula. Use more cooking spray when necessary. Remove from the pan when golden brown in color. Sprinkle lightly with powdered sugar, if using; add whipped topping to taste and garnish with fresh berries.

NUTRITION PER SERVING (2 PANCAKES)

CAL	FAT*	SAT FAT	CHOLEST	SODIUM	CARB	DIET FIBER	SUGARS	PROTEIN
234	16 g	0 g	0 mg	440 mg	35 g	7 g	11 g	9 g

*FAT: 0 g EPA; 0 g DHA; 1 g ALA

From the kitchen of Dr. Janet

CHEF JULIE KORHUMEL'S COLD OATMEAL
WITH YOGURT AND FRESH BERRIES

SERVES 6

1 ½ cups quick-cooking oats

¾ cup fat-free vanilla yogurt, such as Dannon Light & Fit

½ cup orange juice

1 tablespoon honey

¾ cup fresh raspberries

¾ cup diced strawberries

½ cup fresh blueberries

½ medium apple, peeled, cored, and coarsely grated

3 tablespoons ground flaxseeds

¼ cup chopped walnuts

¼ teaspoon ground cinnamon

In a large bowl, combine the oats, yogurt, orange juice, and honey. Let stand for 5 minutes. Gently fold in the raspberries, strawberries, blueberries, apple, flaxseeds, and walnuts. Sprinkle with cinnamon. Cover and refrigerate overnight. Serve cold.

NUTRITION PER ½-CUP SERVING

CAL	FAT*	SAT FAT	CHOLEST	SODIUM	CARB	DIET FIBER	SUGARS	PROTEIN
202	7 g	1 g	1 mg	26 mg	31 g	6 g	12 g	7 g

*FAT: 0 g EPA; 0 g DHA; 2 g ALA

*From the kitchen of
Julie's Gourmet Catering
Libertyville, Illinois*

DR. JANET'S FRESH VEGGIE PITA POCKET SANDWICH

SERVES 1

Quick, tasty, and deliciously healthy.

  1 round 100% whole-wheat pita bread
  2 tablespoons hummus
  ½ cup chopped dark greens
  ¼ cup chopped broccoli florets
  1 tablespoon chopped Vidalia onion
  1 tablespoon diced tomato
  1 tablespoon diced red bell pepper

Cut the pita into two halves. Open the pockets and spread hummus in each pocket. Stuff the veggies evenly inside each pocket and enjoy.

NUTRITION PER SERVING (1 SANDWICH)

CAL	FAT*	SAT FAT	CHOLEST	SODIUM	CARB	DIET FIBER	SUGARS	PROTEIN
235	4 g	1 g	0 mg	485 mg	42 g	5 g	2 g	9 g

*FAT: 0 g EPA; 0 g DHA; 1 g ALA

From the kitchen of Dr. Janet

DR. JANET'S VEGETARIAN
MEXICAN BEAN WRAP SANDWICH

SERVES 1

1 100% whole-wheat tortilla

2 tablespoons canned black beans, drained and rinsed

2 tablespoons frozen corn, thawed

1 tablespoon fat-free shredded Cheddar cheese

¼ cup fat-free salsa

¼ cup chopped fresh spinach

1 slice avocado

Top the tortilla with the beans, corn, and cheese. Microwave on high power for 30 seconds. Roll up with the salsa, spinach, and avocado.

NUTRITION PER SERVING (1 SANDWICH)

CAL	FAT*	SAT FAT	CHOLEST	SODIUM	CARB	DIET FIBER	SUGARS	PROTEIN
228	5 g	0 g	1 mg	465 mg	36 g	5 g	4 g	9 g

*FAT: 0 g EPA; 0 g DHA; 0 g ALA

From the kitchen of Dr. Janet

DR. JANET'S ROASTED RED PEPPER HUMMUS

SERVES 10

Use either jarred red bell peppers or Roasted Red Pepper Strips (page 301) for this tasty dip or sandwich spread. Refrigerate for at least 4 hours for the best flavor.

½ cup roasted red bell pepper strips

One 15-ounce can chickpeas, drained and rinsed

½ cup tahini

2 garlic cloves, minced

Juice of 1 lemon

2 tablespoons extra virgin olive oil

1 teaspoon kosher salt

¼ teaspoon freshly ground black pepper

6 large basil leaves, chopped

In the container of a blender or food processor, mix all of the ingredients with ½ cup water and blend until smooth.

NUTRITION PER ¼-CUP SERVING

CAL	FAT*	SAT FAT	CHOLEST	SODIUM	CARB	DIET FIBER	SUGARS	PROTEIN
141	10 g	1 g	0 mg	243 mg	11 g	3 g	<1 g	4 g

*FAT: 0 g EPA; 0 g DHA; <1 g ALA

From the kitchen of Dr. Janet

CHEF JULIE KORHUMEL'S
CANNELLINI BEAN AND SUN-DRIED TOMATO DIP

SERVES 6

Allow time to refrigerate the dip before serving for the best flavor.

- One 15-ounce can cannellini or great northern beans, drained
- 7 sun-dried tomatoes packed in oil, drained
- 1 garlic clove, peeled and chopped
- ¼ cup extra virgin olive oil
- 2 tablespoons red wine vinegar
- 1 tablespoon chopped fresh rosemary or 1 teaspoon dried
- ½ teaspoon kosher salt
- ½ teaspoon freshly ground black pepper

In the container of a blender or food processor, mix all of the ingredients and blend until smooth. Refrigerate for 1 hour and serve chilled.

NUTRITION PER ¼-CUP SERVING

CAL	FAT*	SAT FAT	CHOLEST	SODIUM	CARB	DIET FIBER	SUGARS	PROTEIN
166	10 g	1 g	0 mg	207 mg	16 g	3 g	<1 g	5 g

*FAT: 0 g EPA; 0 g DHA; <1 g ALA

From the kitchen of
Julie's Gourmet Catering
Libertyville, Illinois

DR. JANET'S BABA GHANOUSH (EGGPLANT DIP)

SERVES 6

Serve cold with Baked Whole-Wheat Pita Chips (page 281).

    1 large eggplant (about 1½ pounds)
    2 garlic cloves, chopped
    ¼ cup chopped flat-leaf parsley
    Juice of 1 lemon
    2 tablespoons extra virgin olive oil
    1 tablespoon tahini
    ¼ teaspoon kosher salt
    ¼ teaspoon cayenne pepper

Preheat the oven to 450°F. Using a fork, prick the eggplant in about eight places. Place on a foil-lined baking sheet. Bake for 35 to 40 minutes, or until soft. Remove from the oven and let cool. Cut the eggplant in half, drain any liquid, and scoop out the pulp into the container of a blender or food processor. Add the garlic, parsley, lemon juice, olive oil, tahini, salt, and cayenne. Blend until smooth. Refrigerate for 30 minutes to blend the flavors.

NUTRITION PER ¼ CUP SERVING

CAL	FAT*	SAT FAT	CHOLEST	SODIUM	CARB	DIET FIBER	SUGARS	PROTEIN
77	6 g	1 g	0 mg	50 mg	6 g	3 g	2 g	1 g

*FAT: 0 g EPA; 0 g DHA; <1 g ALA

From the kitchen of Dr. Janet

CHEF JULIE KORHUMEL'S BASIL PESTO AND TOMATO WHOLE-WHEAT CROSTINI

SERVES 8 (MAKES 16 CROSTINI EACH WITH 1 SLICE BREAD,
1 TEASPOON PESTO, AND 1 GRAPE TOMATO, HALVED)

A beautiful green and red appetizer for a party or premeal starter.

1 cup basil leaves
2 garlic cloves, crushed
¼ cup grated Parmigiano-Reggiano
⅓ cup chopped walnuts
¼ teaspoon kosher salt
¼ teaspoon freshly ground black pepper
½ cup extra virgin olive oil
One 8-ounce whole-wheat baguette, cut into sixteen ½-inch slices
1 cup grape tomatoes, quartered

For pesto:

In the container of a blender or food processor, mix the basil, garlic, cheese, walnuts, salt, and pepper and blend until smooth. With the machine running, slowly add the olive oil to make a thick paste.

For crostini:

Preheat the oven to 350°F. Place the bread slices on a rimmed baking sheet and bake about 12 minutes, until crisp and lightly golden. Remove from the oven and let cool. Spread 1 teaspoon pesto on each slice of bread. Top with the grape tomatoes. Serve immediately.

NUTRITION PER 2-PIECE SERVING

CAL	FAT*	SAT FAT	CHOLEST	SODIUM	CARB	DIET FIBER	SUGARS	PROTEIN
256	19 g	3 g	3 mg	238 mg	18 g	2 g	<1 g	5 g

*FAT: 0 g EPA; 0 g DHA; 1 g ALA

*From the kitchen of
Julie's Gourmet Catering
Libertyville, Illinois*

DR. JANET'S BAKED
WHOLE-WHEAT PITA CHIPS
SERVES 4

Serve these crispy, spicy chips with Roasted Red Pepper Hummus (page 277), Cannellini Bean and Sun-Dried Tomato Dip (page 278), or Baba Ghanoush (page 279).

> 2 tablespoons extra virgin olive oil
>
> 1 teaspoon sesame seeds
>
> ½ teaspoon ground sumac
>
> ½ teaspoon powdered dried thyme
>
> 4 rounds 100% whole-wheat pita bread

Preheat the oven to 350°F. In a small bowl, combine the olive oil, sesame seeds, sumac, and thyme (this is basically the Middle Eastern spice blend za'ata). Brush the oil mixture on the pitas. Bake for 5 minutes on each side. With a large knife, cut each pita into 8 pieces.

NUTRITION PER 8-CHIP SERVING

CAL	FAT*	SAT FAT	CHOLEST	SODIUM	CARB	DIET FIBER	SUGARS	PROTEIN
184	8 g	1 g	0 mg	174 mg	26 g	5 g	<1 g	5 g

*FAT: 0 g EPA; 0 g DHA; <1 g ALA

From the kitchen of Dr. Janet

RACHEL'S TUNA CANNELLINI BEAN SALAD

SERVES 4

A classic combination that is one of my daughter Rachel's favorites. This is for you, my dearest daughter Rachel!

> One 15-ounce can cannellini beans, drained and rinsed
> One 6-ounce can or pouch chunk light tuna packed in water, drained and flaked
> 2 tablespoons finely chopped red onion
> 2 tablespoons chopped fresh basil or sage
> 1 garlic clove, minced
> 2 tablespoons extra virgin olive oil
> Juice of 1 lemon
> ½ teaspoon kosher salt
> ½ teaspoon freshly ground black pepper

In a medium bowl, gently toss the beans and tuna. Fold in the onion, basil, garlic, olive oil, lemon juice, salt, and pepper. Serve immediately or chill until ready to serve.

NUTRITION PER ½-CUP SERVING

CAL	FAT*	SAT FAT	CHOLEST	SODIUM	CARB	DIET FIBER	SUGARS	PROTEIN
244	12 g	3 g	17 mg	422 mg	18 g	4 g	<1 g	17 g

*FAT: O g EPA; O g DHA; <1 g ALA

From the kitchen of Dr. Janet

CHEF JULIE KORHUMEL'S MIXED GREENS WITH LEMON, SHALLOT, AND MUSTARD VINAIGRETTE

SERVES 5

A simple way to dress a fresh bowl of mixed salad greens.

2 tablespoons fresh lemon juice
2 small shallots, minced
2 teaspoons Dijon mustard
½ cup extra virgin olive oil
Kosher salt and freshly ground black pepper
One 5-ounce container mixed salad greens

In a small bowl, whisk the lemon juice, shallots, and mustard. Slowly whisk in the olive oil. Season to taste with salt and pepper. Toss with the mixed salad greens. Serve immediately.

NUTRITION PER SERVING
(1 OUNCE GREENS AND 2 TABLESPOONS VINAIGRETTE)

CAL	FAT*	SAT FAT	CHOLEST	SODIUM	CARB	DIET FIBER	SUGARS	PROTEIN
128	14 g	2 g	0 mg	18 mg	2 g	<1 g	<1 g	1 g

*FAT: 0 g EPA; 0 g DHA; <1 g ALA

From the kitchen of
Julie's Gourmet Catering
Libertyville, Illinois

DR. JANET'S SPINACH SALAD WITH APPLES, TOASTED WALNUTS, AND DRIED CRANBERRIES

SERVES 6

A nice fall dish, rich with spinach, crunchy apples and walnuts, and the sweetness of dried cranberries.

One 5-ounce container baby spinach
2 medium Gala or Braeburn apples, cored and sliced
3 tablespoons extra virgin olive oil
2 tablespoons fresh orange juice
1 teaspoon honey
⅛ teaspoon kosher salt
¼ teaspoon freshly ground black pepper
¼ cup chopped walnuts, toasted
2 tablespoons dried cranberries

Arrange the spinach on a large platter or in a large, shallow salad bowl. Top with the sliced apples. In a small bowl, mix the olive oil, orange juice, honey, salt, and pepper. Drizzle over the spinach and apples. Sprinkle with the walnuts and cranberries. Serve immediately.

NUTRITION PER 1½-CUP SERVING

CAL	FAT*	SAT FAT	CHOLEST	SODIUM	CARB	DIET FIBER	SUGARS	PROTEIN
139	10 g	1 g	0 mg	49 mg	13 g	2 g	9 g	2 g

*FAT: 0 g EPA; 0 g DHA; 1 g ALA

From the kitchen of Dr. Janet

DR. JANET'S ARUGULA SALAD WITH FIGS AND WALNUTS

SERVES 6

The peppery bite of arugula blends well with the soft flavor of the figs.

> One 5-ounce container baby arugula
> ¼ cup Parsley Chive Dressing (page 288)
> 1 cup chopped dried Mission figs
> ½ cup chopped walnuts, toasted

In a large bowl toss the arugula with the Parsley Chive Dressing. Arrange the arugula on a platter or in a shallow bowl. Sprinkle with the figs and walnuts. Serve with more dressing on the side, if desired.

NUTRITION PER SERVING (1¼ CUPS ARUGULA AND 2 TEASPOONS DRESSING)

CAL	FAT*	SAT FAT	CHOLEST	SODIUM	CARB	DIET FIBER	SUGARS	PROTEIN
173	11 g	1 g	0 mg	15 mg	18 g	4 g	13 g	3 g

*FAT: 0 g EPA; 0 g DHA; 1 g ALA

From the kitchen of Dr. Janet

CHEF JULIE KORHUMEL'S GREEK SALAD

SERVES 5

Bright and colorful, best made with garden-fresh vegetables.

> 1 medium cucumber, peeled, seeded, cut in half lengthwise, and sliced
> 1 large ripe tomato, cut in half and sliced
> ⅓ cup thinly sliced red onion
> ½ cup pitted Kalamata olives, cut in half
> ⅓ cup crumbled fat-free feta cheese
> Juice of ½ lemon
> 1 tablespoon extra virgin olive oil
> 2 teaspoons red wine vinegar
> Kosher salt and freshly ground black pepper
> ⅓ cup thinly sliced basil

In a medium bowl, layer the cucumber, tomato, onion, olives, and cheese. In a separate bowl, whisk the lemon juice, olive oil, and vinegar. Season to taste with salt and pepper. Pour the dressing over the salad and garnish with the basil.

NUTRITION PER 1-CUP SERVING

CAL	FAT*	SAT FAT	CHOLEST	SODIUM	CARB	DIET FIBER	SUGARS	PROTEIN
61	4 g	1 g	1 mg	220 mg	5 g	2 g	2 g	2 g

*FAT: 0 g EPA; 0 g DHA; <1 g ALA

From the kitchen of
Julie's Gourmet Catering
Libertyville, Illinois

CHEF KERN MATTEI'S APPLE CARROT SALAD

SERVES 4

A nice side salad served with Pan-Seared Salmon (page 321).

- 1 tablespoon reduced-sodium soy sauce
- 1 tablespoon fresh lime juice
- ½ teaspoon sugar
- 1 Granny Smith apple, cored and julienned
- 1 large carrot, julienned
- 3 cilantro sprigs, chopped

In a small bowl, mix the soy sauce, lime juice, and sugar until the sugar is dissolved. In a medium bowl, gently toss the apple, carrot, and cilantro with the dressing.

NUTRITION PER ½-CUP SERVING

CAL	FAT*	SAT FAT	CHOLEST.	SODIUM	CARB	DIET FIBER	SUGARS	PROTEIN
27	<1 g	<1 g	0 mg	44 mg	7 g	1 g	5 g	<1 g

*FAT: 0 g EPA; 0 g DHA; <1 g ALA

From the kitchen of
Mai-Kai Restaurant
3599 North Federal Highway
Fort Lauderdale, Florida

DR. JANET'S PARSLEY CHIVE DRESSING

SERVES 12

Delicious served on a salad or a fillet of Grilled Swordfish (page 319), or Pan-Seared Salmon (page 321).

> ¾ cup extra virgin olive oil
> ¼ cup aged balsamic vinegar
> 1 tablespoon Dijon mustard
> 1 shallot, minced
> 1 bunch flat-leaf parsley, stalks removed
> 3 stalks fresh chives, cut into small pieces

Place all of the ingredients in the container of a blender. Blend until the ingredients are well combined, scraping down the sides of the container at least once.

NUTRITION PER 2-TABLESPOON SERVING

CAL	FAT*	SAT FAT	CHOLEST	SODIUM	CARB	DIET FIBER	SUGARS	PROTEIN
123	14 g	2 g	0 mg	18 mg	1 g	<1 g	<1 g	<1 g

*FAT: 0 g EPA; 0 g DHA; <1 g ALA

From the kitchen of Dr. Janet

CHEF MARIO SPINA'S GREEN PEA AND LIMA BEAN SOUP
SERVES 8

Surprisingly easy and made from readily available ingredients.

> ¼ cup extra virgin olive oil, plus more for garnish
> 1 large sweet onion, chopped
> One 1-pound bag frozen green peas
> One 1-pound bag frozen baby lima beans
> 1 teaspoon kosher salt
> ½ teaspoon freshly ground black pepper
> 8 cups reduced-sodium chicken broth or water

In a soup pot, heat ¼ cup olive oil over medium heat. Add the onion and cook until golden brown, 10 to 12 minutes. Stir in the peas and lima beans. Cook, stirring occasionally, for 10 minutes. Stir in the broth, bring to a boil, and reduce to a simmer. Cook until the peas and beans are soft, about 20 minutes. In the container of a blender or food processor, purée the soup until velvety. Season with salt and pepper. Serve each bowl drizzled with olive oil.

NUTRITION PER 1-CUP SERVING

CAL	FAT*	SAT FAT	CHOLEST	SODIUM	CARB	DIET FIBER	SUGARS	PROTEIN
201	7 g	1 g	0 mg	791 mg	25 g	6 g	4 g	10 g

*FAT: 0 g EPA; 0 g DHA; <1 g ALA

From the kitchen of
Mario Ristorante Italiano and Wine Bar
6370 North State Road 7
Coconut Creek, Florida

CHEF JULIE KORHUMEL'S
ROASTED FRESH TOMATO SOUP

SERVES 6

For the best flavor, use fresh, ripe tomatoes. Roasting brings out the natural sweetness in the tomato and the onion. Good served hot or cold.

> Nonstick cooking spray
> 3½ pounds ripe tomatoes, halved
> 1 small onion, quartered
> 2 garlic cloves, halved
> 2 tablespoons extra virgin olive oil
> 2 tablespoons fresh thyme
> 1 teaspoon kosher salt
> ¼ teaspoon freshly ground black pepper
> 15 basil leaves

Preheat the oven to 400°F. Spray a large rimmed baking sheet with nonstick cooking spray. Place the tomatoes, onion, and garlic on the prepared pan. Drizzle with the olive oil, thyme, ½ teaspoon salt, and pepper. Shake the pan back and forth a few times to coat the vegetables with the oil and seasonings. Bake until tender, about 25 minutes. When cool, blend the roasted tomatoes and onion, along with the basil and the remaining ½ teaspoon salt, in batches if necessary. Transfer to a saucepan and heat if desired, or refrigerate to chill.

NUTRITION PER 1-CUP SERVING

CAL	FAT*	SAT FAT	CHOLEST	SODIUM	CARB	DIET FIBER	SUGARS	PROTEIN
135	10 g	1 g	0 mg	208 mg	12 g	4 g	7 g	3 g

*FAT: 0 g EPA; 0 g DHA; <1 g ALA

From the kitchen of
Julie's Gourmet Catering
Libertyville, Illinois

CHEF JULIE KORHUMEL'S LENTIL SOUP

SERVES 9

A beautiful soup, full of fiber-rich lentils and finished with fresh herbs.

1½ tablespoons extra virgin olive oil

1½ large onions, diced (about 2 cups)

5 carrots, diced (about 2 cups)

4 garlic cloves, chopped

2 cups brown lentils, rinsed and picked over

One 15-ounce can diced tomatoes

¼ cup tomato paste

1 tablespoon curry powder

1 tablespoon sweet paprika

1 cup chopped fresh parsley

1 cup chopped fresh cilantro

1 extra-large vegetarian bouillon cube, such as Knorr's

½ teaspoon Tabasco sauce

In a large soup pot, heat the olive oil over medium heat. Add the onions, carrots, and garlic and cook until softened and golden, about 10 minutes. Stir in the lentils, tomatoes, tomato paste, curry powder, paprika, and 6 cups water. Cook until the lentils are soft, stirring frequently, about 30 minutes. Add the parsley, cilantro, bouillon cube, and Tabasco, stirring to dissolve the bouillon cube. Serve hot.

NUTRITION PER 1-CUP SERVING

CAL	FAT*	SAT FAT	CHOLEST	SODIUM	CARB	DIET FIBER	SUGARS	PROTEIN
212	3 g	<1 g	0 mg	150 mg	35 g	16 g	7 g	14 g

*FAT: 0 g EPA; 0 g DHA; <1 g ALA

From the kitchen of
Julie's Gourmet Catering
Libertyville, Illinois

DR. JANET'S WHOLE-GRAIN PASTA WITH ROASTED EGGPLANT, OLIVES, AND TOMATOES

SERVES 8

Roasting the tomatoes and eggplant adds a sweet, rich flavor to the vegetables. Delicious served with whole-grain pasta.

Nonstick cooking spray
2 pints grape tomatoes
One 1½-pound eggplant, cut into 1-inch cubes
1 cup pitted Kalamata olives
6 garlic cloves, roughly chopped
¼ cup extra virgin olive oil
2 tablespoons fresh thyme leaves or 2 teaspoons dried
1 teaspoon kosher salt
1 teaspoon crushed red pepper flakes
½ cup thinly sliced basil
1 cup Roasted Red Pepper Strips (page 301)
4 cups (about 8 ounces) whole-grain rotini or penne pasta

Preheat the oven to 375°F. Spray a rimmed baking sheet with nonstick cooking spray. Place the tomatoes, eggplant cubes, olives, and garlic on the prepared baking sheet. Drizzle with the olive oil and season with the thyme, salt, and red pepper flakes. Shake the baking sheet back and forth a few times to coat the vegetables with the oil and seasonings. Roast for 1 hour 10 minutes, until the tomatoes are softened and the eggplant is lightly browned. When the vegetables are done, remove them from the oven and spoon them into a shallow bowl or platter. Stir in the basil and Roasted Red Pepper Strips. Near the end of the cooking time, bring a large pot of water to a boil. Add the pasta and cook until al dente, about 10 minutes. Serve the vegetables over the hot whole-grain pasta.

NUTRITION PER SERVING (½ CUP SAUCE AND ½ CUP DRY PASTA)

CAL	FAT*	SAT FAT	CHOLEST	SODIUM	CARB	DIET FIBER	SUGARS	PROTEIN
249	13 g	2 g	0 mg	364 mg	32 g	5 g	5 g	6 g

*FAT: 0 g EPA; 0 g DHA; <1 g ALA

From the kitchen of Dr. Janet

CHEF JULIE KORHUMEL'S
LINGUINE WITH FRESH GARDEN VEGETABLES

SERVES 8

Delicious served hot or cold.

8 ounces whole-wheat linguine, cooked
½ red bell pepper, seeded and thinly sliced
1½ cups fresh spinach, roughly chopped
¾ cup sugar snap peas, sliced lengthwise
¾ cup grape tomatoes, halved
½ cup chopped fresh basil
¼ cup chopped scallion
⅓ cup extra virgin olive oil
Juice of 1 lemon
1 garlic clove, minced
1 tablespoon white balsamic vinegar
½ teaspoon kosher salt
Freshly ground black pepper
¼ cup shaved Parmigiano-Reggiano

Bring a large pot of water to a boil. Add the linguine and cook until al dente, about 10 minutes. Drain and rinse. In a large bowl, toss the linguine with the bell pepper, spinach, peas, tomatoes, basil, and scallion. In a medium bowl, whisk the olive oil, lemon juice, garlic, vinegar, salt, and pepper together until thick. Toss with the linguine and vegetables. Serve with shaved cheese on top.

NUTRITION PER SERVING (⅛ RECIPE)

CAL	FAT*	SAT FAT	CHOLEST	SODIUM	CARB	DIET FIBER	SUGARS	PROTEIN
132	10 g	1 g	1 mg	101 mg	11 g	2 g	1 g	3 g

*FAT: 0 g EPA; 0 g DHA; <1 g ALA

From the kitchen of
Julie's Gourmet Catering
Libertyville, Illinois

CHEF KEITH BLAUSCHILD'S
HERBED RED BEANS AND BROWN RICE

SERVES 4

A tea bag steeped in the cooking liquid adds a beautiful brown hue to the rice.

  1¾ cups reduced-sodium chicken broth or water
  1 black tea bag
  ¾ cup long-grain brown rice
  1 tablespoon extra virgin olive oil
  1 tablespoon chopped garlic
  One 16-ounce can red beans or kidney beans, undrained (about 2 cups)
  ¼ cup tomato paste
  1 tablespoon chopped fresh oregano
  Pinch of crushed red pepper flakes
  ¼ cup minced fresh parsley
  ¼ cup chopped scallion

In a medium saucepan, bring the broth to a boil over medium heat. Add the tea bag and boil for 30 seconds. Remove the tea bag and stir in the rice. Bring to a simmer, cover, reduce the heat to low and cook for 40 minutes. Meanwhile, in a large skillet, heat the olive oil over medium heat. Add the garlic and cook until golden, about 2 minutes. Add the beans, tomato paste, oregano, and red pepper flakes. Reduce the heat to low and simmer for 15 to 20 minutes, until the sauce is thickened. Stir in the parsley and scallion and serve over the hot brown rice.

NUTRITION PER SERVING (½ CUP BEANS AND 1⅓ CUPS COOKED RICE)

CAL	FAT*	SAT FAT	CHOLEST	SODIUM	CARB	DIET FIBER	SUGARS	PROTEIN
342	11 g	3 g	6 mg	651 mg	50 g	7 g	2 g	13 g

*FAT: 0 g EPA; 0 g DHA; <1 g ALA

From the kitchen of
Parkland Chef Catering
2151 Riverside Drive
Coral Springs, Florida

DR. JANET'S WHOLE-GRAIN ROTINI
WITH RATATOUILLE
SERVES 6

The ratatouille can be made up to 2 days ahead, if desired, to allow the flavors to expand.

- 4 tablespoons extra virgin olive oil
- 2 large onions, chopped
- 2 garlic cloves, minced
- 2 red bell peppers, seeded and chopped
- 1½ pounds zucchini (about 4 small), cut in half lengthwise and sliced
- 2 tablespoons fresh thyme or 2 teaspoons dried
- 1 tablespoon chopped fresh oregano or 1 teaspoon dried
- 1 tablespoon chopped fresh basil or 1 teaspoon dried
- 2 bay leaves
- 1 teaspoon kosher salt
- ½ teaspoon freshly ground black pepper
- 2 large tomatoes, diced
- ¼ cup chopped fresh basil, optional
- 3 cups (about 6 ounces) whole-wheat rotini

In a Dutch oven, heat 2 tablespoons olive oil over medium heat. Add the onions and cook until softened, about 5 minutes. Stir in the garlic and bell peppers and cook for 5 more minutes. Add the zucchini, thyme, oregano, basil, bay leaves, salt, and pepper. Stir well to combine and cook for 10 minutes. Add the tomatoes and bring to a simmer. Partially cover, reduce the heat to low, and cook for 30 minutes. Stir in 2 tablespoons olive oil and the fresh basil, if using. Meanwhile, bring a large pot of water to a boil. Add the rotini and cook until al dente, about 10 minutes. Heat the ratatouille, if needed, remove the bay leaves, and serve over the rotini.

NUTRITION PER SERVING (1 CUP RATATOUILLE AND ½ CUP DRY PASTA)

CAL	FAT*	SAT FAT	CHOLEST	SODIUM	CARB	DIET FIBER	SUGARS	PROTEIN
234	10 g	1 g	0 mg	213 mg	34 g	3 g	6 g	7 g

*FAT: 0 g EPA; 0 g DHA; <1 g ALA

From the kitchen of Dr. Janet

CHEF KEITH BLAUSCHILD'S CHICKPEAS WITH ROASTED PEPPERS AND ORANGE ZEST

SERVES 4

A nice, warm side dish, flavored with the essence of orange and cumin.

> One 15-ounce can chickpeas
> Zest of 1 orange
> Juice of 1 orange
> ½ cup chopped roasted red bell pepper
> ¼ cup chopped fresh cilantro
> ½ teaspoon ground cumin
> ¼ teaspoon kosher salt

Drain the chickpeas, reserving ¼ cup liquid. Place the chickpeas and orange zest in a serving bowl. In a small saucepan over low heat, warm the ¼ cup reserved chickpea liquid and orange juice until steaming. Turn off the heat and mix in the bell pepper, cilantro, cumin, and salt. Pour over the chickpeas. Serve warm.

NUTRITION PER ½-CUP SERVING

CAL	FAT*	SAT FAT	CHOLEST	SODIUM	CARB	DIET FIBER	SUGARS	PROTEIN
163	6 g	2 g	4 mg	331 mg	21 g	5 g	2 g	6 g

*FAT: 0 g EPA; 0 g DHA; 0 g ALA

From the kitchen of
Parkland Chef Catering
2151 Riverside Drive
Coral Springs, Florida

DR. JESSICA FRISK'S RED LENTIL CURRY

SERVES 8

Jessica is our longtime Swedish family friend who is not only a great cook but a talented surgeon as well. Here is her delicious version of red lentil curry, one which in her own words "surely prevents diverticulitis!"

2 tablespoons extra virgin olive oil
1 medium white onion, diced
2 medium red potatoes, diced
2 carrots, diced
1 red bell pepper, seeded and chopped
2 garlic cloves, chopped
1 tablespoon curry powder
1 teaspoon paprika
1 teaspoon ground cinnamon
1 teaspoon chili powder
1 cup red lentils, rinsed
3 cups reduced-sodium chicken broth
1 medium Granny Smith or Golden Delicious apple, cored and diced
1 tablespoon brown sugar
Pinch of cocoa powder
½ teaspoon kosher salt

In a large skillet, heat the olive oil over medium heat. Add the onion, potatoes, carrots, bell pepper, and garlic and cook until the onion is lightly browned, about 8 minutes. Add the curry powder, paprika, cinnamon, and chili powder and stir to combine. Add the lentils and broth and simmer, covered, until the carrots and lentils are soft, about 20 minutes. Stir in the apple, brown sugar, cocoa powder, and salt and simmer, covered, for about 10 minutes, until the apples are soft. Serve warm.

NUTRITION PER 1-CUP SERVING

CAL	FAT*	SAT FAT	CHOLEST	SODIUM	CARB	DIET FIBER	SUGARS	PROTEIN
195	4 g	1 g	0 mg	374 mg	32 g	5 g	6 g	9 g

*FAT: 0 g EPA; 0 g DHA; <1 g ALA

From the kitchen of Dr. Jessica Frisk

MIA'S WHOLE-GRAIN PIZZA WITH ARUGULA, EGGPLANT, AND CARAMELIZED ONION

MAKES 16 SLICES

This recipe makes two 12-inch pizzas. One pound of store-bought whole-wheat pizza dough made with olive oil can be substituted for homemade dough, if desired. If King Arthur flour is not available in your area, substitute 1 cup whole-wheat flour mixed with 1¾ cups unbleached all-purpose flour. This is for you, my dearest daughter Mia, who loves pizza!

DOUGH:

2¾ cups King Arthur white whole-wheat flour

2 tablespoons quick-rising yeast

1 teaspoon kosher salt

1 cup warm water (105° to 115°F)

¼ cup extra virgin olive oil

½ teaspoon honey

Nonstick cooking spray

In the container of a food processor fitted with a plastic blade, blend the flour, yeast, and salt. In a 2-cup measuring cup, mix the water, olive oil, and honey. With the food processor running, add the water-oil mixture and blend until the flour forms a ball of dough. Process for 1 minute to knead the dough. The dough will be a bit sticky, but if it is too wet, add up to ½ cup more flour. Spray a bowl with nonstick cooking spray. Put the dough into the prepared bowl, cover with plastic wrap, and let rise in a warm place until the dough is doubled in size, about 1 hour.

TOPPINGS:

⅜ cup extra virgin olive oil

2 large onions, thinly sliced

1¼ teaspoons kosher salt

¼ teaspoon freshly ground black pepper

One 8-ounce eggplant, cut into 1-inch cubes

5 ounces (about 4 cups) baby arugula

2 teaspoons cornmeal

¼ cup finely shredded Parmigiano-Reggiano

In a large skillet over medium heat, heat 2 tablespoons olive oil. Add the onions, ½ the salt, and pepper. Cook, stirring occasionally until golden brown, about 15 minutes. Remove to a bowl. In the same skillet, heat 1 tablespoon olive oil. Add the eggplant and remaining salt and cook, stirring, for 2 minutes. Cover and cook, stirring occasionally, for 5 minutes to soften the eggplant. Uncover and cook for 2 to 3 more minutes to remove any excess moisture. Remove to a bowl. In the same skillet, heat 1 tablespoon olive oil. Add the arugula and cook, tossing the arugula until it is wilted. Remove from the skillet and set aside.

To assemble the pizzas, preheat the oven, and a baking stone if desired, to 425°F. Punch down the dough and divide into two pieces. Set on a lightly floured surface and cover with a towel to rest for 5 minutes. For each pizza, sprinkle a baking sheet with 1 teaspoon cornmeal. Roll one piece of dough into a 12-inch circle and place on the prepared baking sheet. Brush the dough with 1 tablespoon olive oil. Distribute ½ cup caramelized onions, ½ cup cooked eggplant, and ¼ cup arugula on the dough. Sprinkle each pizza with 2 tablespoons shredded cheese. Bake the pizzas for about 15 minutes, until the crust is lightly browned. Cut each pizza into 8 slices.

NUTRITION PER SERVING (1 SLICE OF PIZZA)

CAL	FAT*	SAT FAT	CHOLEST	SODIUM	CARB	DIET FIBER	SUGARS	PROTEIN
164	9 g	1 g	1 mg	335 mg	18 g	4 g	1 g	4 g

*FAT: 0 g EPA; 0 g DHA; <1 g ALA

From the kitchen of Dr. Janet

JASON'S SLOW COOKER TURKEY AND BEAN CHILI

SERVES 6

This is my son's favorite dish, so this is for you, my dearest Jason! Serve warm over brown rice and garnished with a touch of shredded soy Cheddar cheese.

> 2 tablespoons extra virgin olive oil
> 4 garlic cloves, sliced
> 1¼ pounds extra-lean ground turkey breast
> Nonstick cooking spray
> Two 26.46-ounce containers no-salt-added Pomi chopped tomatoes
> Two 16-ounce cans dark red kidney beans, drained and rinsed
> One 15-ounce can black beans, drained and rinsed
> ½ medium onion, chopped
> 1 cup frozen corn, thawed
> 2 tablespoons chili powder
> 1 teaspoon crushed red pepper flakes
> ½ tablespoon garlic powder
> ½ tablespoon ground cumin
> Pinch of freshly ground black pepper
> Pinch of ground allspice
> Kosher salt, optional

In a large skillet over medium-high heat, heat the olive oil and garlic until the garlic is light golden brown. Place the turkey in the skillet and cook until evenly browned. Coat the inside of a slow cooker with nonstick cooking spray. Mix the turkey, tomatoes, kidney beans, black beans, onion, and corn. Season with the chili powder, red pepper flakes, garlic powder, cumin, pepper, allspice (kosher salt if desired), and blend. Cover and cook for 4 hours on high (or 8 hours on low).

NUTRITION PER 1-CUP SERVING

CAL	FAT*	SAT FAT	CHOLEST	SODIUM	CARB	DIET FIBER	SUGARS	PROTEIN
356	6 g	1 g	2 mg	29 mg	59 g	21 g	11 g	19 g

*FAT: O g EPA; O g DHA; O g ALA

From the kitchen of Dr. Janet

DR. JANET'S ROASTED RED PEPPER STRIPS
SERVES 4

A quick and easy method for roasting red peppers. Delicious in Roasted Red Pepper Hummus (page 277), Tuna Romesco (page 324), and Whole-Grain Pasta with Roasted Eggplant, Olives, and Tomatoes (page 292).

> 4 large red bell peppers, seeded and cut into ½-inch-thick strips
> 3 tablespoons extra virgin olive oil
> 1 teaspoon kosher salt
> ½ teaspoon freshly ground black pepper

Preheat the oven to 375° F. Toss the bell pepper strips with the olive oil, salt, and pepper. Spread on a rimmed baking sheet and bake for about 50 minutes, or until the peppers are softened and starting to turn dark around the edges. Store refrigerated.

NUTRITION PER ½-CUP SERVING

CAL	FAT*	SAT FAT	CHOLEST	SODIUM	CARB	DIET FIBER	SUGARS	PROTEIN
133	11 g	1 g	0 mg	294 mg	10 g	3 g	7 g	2 g

*FAT: 0 g EPA; 0 g DHA; <1 g ALA

From the kitchen of Dr. Janet

CHEF MARIO SPINA'S BRAISED BROCCOLI RABE

SERVES 4

The secret to bright green broccoli rabe, without a hint of bitterness, is precooking it in boiling water and cooling it for up to 1 hour in an ice-water bath.

   2 bunches broccoli rabe
   ½ teaspoon kosher salt, plus more to taste
   2 tablespoons extra virgin olive oil
   4 garlic cloves, chopped
   ¼ teaspoon crushed red pepper flakes

Trim the broccoli rabe and chop it into 2-inch pieces. In a large pot, bring 4 quarts water and ½ teaspoon salt to a boil. Drop the broccoli rabe into the boiling water and cook for 3 minutes. Drain and cool in ice water for 30 minutes to 1 hour. Drain well. In a large skillet, heat the olive oil over medium-high heat. Add the garlic and red pepper flakes and cook for several minutes until the garlic is golden brown. Add the broccoli rabe, cover, and reduce the heat to medium low. Cook for 4 minutes to heat the broccoli rabe. Toss with salt to taste just before serving.

NUTRITION PER ½-BUNCH SERVING

CAL	FAT*	SAT FAT	CHOLEST	SODIUM	CARB	DIET FIBER	SUGARS	PROTEIN
92	8 g	1 g	0 mg	112 mg	5 g	3 g	<1 g	4 g

*FAT: 0 g EPA; 0 g DHA; <1 g ALA

From the kitchen of
Mario Ristorante Italiano and Wine Bar
6370 North State Road 7
Coconut Creek, Florida

CHEF KERN MATTEI'S PEA PODS
WITH ALMONDS
SERVES 4

Fresh pea pods only need to be washed and trimmed before cooking and can be eaten pods and all. They are perfect for stir-fry dishes, because their tender sweet crispness needs little cooking. For this dish, have all ingredients ready before cooking, because it cooks very fast.

    1 tablespoon extra virgin olive oil
    2 garlic cloves, sliced
    2 cups sugar snap pea pods, trimmed
    1 teaspoon dry white wine, such as Chardonnay
    ¼ teaspoon kosher salt
    ¼ teaspoon sugar
    ¼ cup sliced almonds, toasted

Heat a large skillet over medium-high heat. Add the olive oil and when it is very hot, add the garlic. Cook, stirring constantly, for 4 to 5 seconds. Add the pea pods and cook, stirring, for another 15 to 20 seconds. Add the wine, salt, and sugar and continue to cook while stirring constantly for another 20 seconds. Sprinkle with the almonds, mix well, and serve immediately.

NUTRITION PER ½-CUP SERVING

CAL	FAT*	SAT FAT	CHOLEST	SODIUM	CARB	DIET FIBER	SUGARS	PROTEIN
80	6 g	1 g	0 mg	72 mg	5 g	2 g	2 g	2 g

*FAT: 0 g EPA; 0 g DHA; <1 g ALA

From the kitchen of
Mai-Kai Restaurant
3599 North Federal Highway
Fort Lauderdale, Florida

DR. JANET'S ROASTED BRUSSELS SPROUTS

SERVES 4

When roasted with slices of fresh garlic, Brussels sprouts turn into a vegetable everyone will love.

    1 pound Brussels sprouts, trimmed and halved
    2 tablespoons extra virgin olive oil
    3 garlic cloves, sliced
    ½ teaspoon kosher salt
    ½ teaspoon freshly ground black pepper

Preheat the oven to 375° F. In a glass baking dish, toss the Brussels sprouts with the olive oil, garlic, salt, and pepper. Bake for 30 to 35 minutes, until lightly browned.

NUTRITION PER ⅔-CUP SERVING

CAL	FAT*	SAT FAT	CHOLEST	SODIUM	CARB	DIET FIBER	SUGARS	PROTEIN
113	7 g	1 g	0 mg	174 mg	11 g	4 g	3 g	4 g

*FAT: 0 g EPA; 0 g DHA; <1 g ALA

From the kitchen of Dr. Janet

DR. JANET'S ROASTED BEETS
WITH LEMON VINAIGRETTE
SERVES 6

Earthy beets are a beautiful side dish when roasted, peeled, and topped with a lemony vinaigrette and fresh parsley.

    Nonstick cooking spray
    6 beets, trimmed of greens and roots
    2 tablespoons extra virgin olive oil
    2 teaspoons fresh lemon juice
    1 garlic clove, minced
    1 teaspoon Dijon mustard
    ¼ teaspoon kosher salt
    ¼ teaspoon freshly ground black pepper
    ¼ cup chopped flat-leaf parsley

Spray a baking dish with nonstick cooking spray. Place the beets in the dish and cover tightly with foil. Bake the beets for about 1 hour, or until they are tender when pierced with a fork or thin knife. Remove from the oven and allow to cool to the touch. Meanwhile, in a small bowl, whisk the olive oil, lemon juice, garlic, mustard, salt, and pepper for the dressing. When the beets are cool enough to handle, peel and slice the beets, arranging the slices on a platter. Drizzle with the vinaigrette and garnish with parsley.

NUTRITION PER SERVING (EACH BEET AND 1 TEASPOON VINAIGRETTE)

CAL	FAT*	SAT FAT	CHOLEST	SODIUM	CARB	DIET FIBER	SUGARS	PROTEIN
69	6 g	1 g	0 mg	222 mg	4 g	1 g	<1 g	1 g

*FAT: 0 g EPA; 0 g DHA; <1 g ALA

From the kitchen of Dr. Janet

DR. JANET'S ROASTED CAULIFLOWER
WITH PINE NUTS AND TARRAGON
SERVES 8

This is a favorite: fresh roasted cauliflower turned into a warm side dish with fresh tarragon and toasted pine nuts.

> 1 medium head (about 1½ pounds) cauliflower, cut into 1-inch florets
> ¼ cup plus 2 tablespoons extra virgin olive oil
> ½ teaspoon kosher salt
> ½ teaspoon freshly ground black pepper
> ⅓ cup raisins
> 2 tablespoons red wine vinegar
> 2 garlic cloves, minced
> 1 tablespoon grainy brown mustard
> 1 tablespoon chopped fresh tarragon
> ⅓ cup pine nuts, toasted

Preheat the oven to 350°F. Spread the cauliflower on a rimmed baking sheet. Drizzle with 2 tablespoons olive oil and sprinkle with salt and pepper. Gently shake the sheet back and forth to coat the cauliflower in olive oil. Bake for 30 to 35 minutes, until lightly browned around the edges. Meanwhile, in a serving bowl, soak the raisins in the vinegar for 10 minutes. Mix in the garlic, mustard, tarragon, and ¼ cup olive oil to make a dressing. When the cauliflower is done, place the roasted florets in the bowl and toss with the dressing. Sprinkle with the pine nuts. Serve warm.

NUTRITION PER ½-CUP SERVING

CAL	FAT*	SAT FAT	CHOLEST	SODIUM	CARB	DIET FIBER	SUGARS	PROTEIN
167	14 g	2 g	0 mg	82 mg	10 g	2 g	6 g	3 g

*FAT: 0 g EPA; 0 g DHA; <1 g ALA

From the kitchen of Dr. Janet

DR. JANET'S BRAISED
RED CABBAGE WITH GREEN OLIVES

SERVES 6

A quick and easy way to enjoy the beautiful color of fresh red cabbage.

- 1½-pound head red cabbage
- 2 tablespoons extra virgin olive oil
- 1 tablespoon red wine vinegar
- ½ cup chopped green olives
- ¼ cup capers
- ½ teaspoon kosher salt
- ½ teaspoon freshly ground black pepper

Remove the outer leaves from the cabbage and slice it into ¼-inch strips, discarding the core. In a Dutch oven, heat the olive oil over medium-high heat. Add the cabbage and cook, stirring, for 5 minutes. Stir in 2 tablespoons water and the vinegar. Cover and cook for 5 more minutes. Stir in the olives, capers, salt, and pepper.

NUTRITION PER SERVING (⅔ CUP CABBAGE)

CAL	FAT*	SAT FAT	CHOLEST	SODIUM	CARB	DIET FIBER	SUGARS	PROTEIN
90	6 g	1 g	0 mg	513 mg	9 g	3 g	4 g	2 g

*FAT: 0 g EPA; 0 g DHA; <1 g ALA

From the kitchen of Dr. Janet

DR. JANET'S OVEN-ROASTED RED POTATOES

SERVES 6

Herbes de Provence is a mix of dried herbs reflecting those most commonly used in southern France. Lavender, marjoram, sage, thyme, and sometimes fennel seeds make this herb blend unique and an elegant way to season vegetables.

1½ pounds small red potatoes, quartered
2 tablespoons extra virgin olive oil
2 teaspoons herbes de Provence
1 teaspoon kosher salt
1 teaspoon freshly ground black pepper
½ cup sliced Kalamata olives
¼ cup chopped fresh parsley

Preheat the oven to 400°F. In a large bowl, toss the potatoes with the olive oil, herbes de Provence, salt, and pepper. Place the potatoes in a single layer on a rimmed baking sheet, cut side down. Bake for 35 to 40 minutes, until the potatoes are soft when pierced with a fork and browned. When the potatoes are cooked, remove them from the baking sheet and place on a platter. Toss with the olives and parsley. Serve warm.

NUTRITION PER SERVING (⅔ CUP POTATOES)

CAL	FAT*	SAT FAT	CHOLEST	SODIUM	CARB	DIET FIBER	SUGARS	PROTEIN
143	6 g	1 g	0 mg	469 mg	21 g	3 g	1 g	3 g

*FAT: 0 g EPA; 0 g DHA; <1 g ALA

From the kitchen of Dr. Janet

DR. JANET'S SPINACH
WITH PINE NUTS AND RAISINS

SERVES 2

A quick, easy, and most delicious way to serve fresh spinach.

- 2 tablespoons pine nuts
- 1 tablespoon extra virgin olive oil
- 2 garlic cloves, sliced
- 2 tablespoons raisins
- One 5-ounce container baby spinach
- ¼ teaspoon kosher salt
- ½ teaspoon freshly ground black pepper

In a large skillet, carefully toast the pine nuts over medium heat until lightly browned. Remove the pine nuts to a dish. In the same skillet, heat the olive oil over medium heat. Add the garlic and raisins and stir while cooking to soften, about 1 minute. Stir in the spinach. Using a pair of tongs or two wooden spoons, toss the spinach with the oil to wilt the spinach. Turn off the heat and season with the salt and pepper. Sprinkle with the pine nuts and serve immediately.

NUTRITION PER SCANT 1-CUP SERVING

CAL	FAT*	SAT FAT	CHOLEST	SODIUM	CARB	DIET FIBER	SUGARS	PROTEIN
166	13 g	1 g	0 mg	128 mg	13 g	2 g	6 g	4 g

*FAT: 0 g EPA; 0 g DHA; <1 g ALA

From the kitchen of Dr. Janet

SAM'S PORTOBELLO PIZZAS

SERVES 6

Basil pesto makes a pretty and delicious topping for these pizzas. This pizza is a favorite of my husband, Sam, so this is for you, my dearest Sam!

6 portobello mushrooms, stems removed and brushed clean
2 tablespoons Basil Pesto (page 280)
2 tablespoons fat-free feta cheese
1½ teaspoons chopped garlic
½ cup halved Kalamata olives
½ teaspoon kosher salt
½ teaspoon freshly ground black pepper

Preheat the oven to 375° F. Place the mushroom caps on a rimmed baking sheet, gill side up. Bake for 5 minutes. Remove from the oven and spread 1 teaspoon Basil Pesto on each mushroom. Top each cap with 1 teaspoon cheese, ¼ teaspoon garlic, and 6 to 8 olive halves, and sprinkle with salt and pepper. Bake for 20 minutes, until the mushrooms are softened and the cheese melts. Serve hot.

NUTRITION PER 1-MUSHROOM SERVING

CAL	FAT*	SAT FAT	CHOLEST	SODIUM	CARB	DIET FIBER	SUGARS	PROTEIN
67	5 g	1 g	5 mg	222 mg	4 g	1 g	1 g	3 g

*FAT: 0 g EPA; 0 g DHA; <1 g ALA

From the kitchen of Dr. Janet

DR. JANET'S BARLEY MUSHROOM PILAF

SERVES 8

This hearty grain, paired with sautéed mushrooms and onions, makes a fiber-rich side dish.

2 tablespoons extra virgin olive oil

½ medium onion, finely chopped

1 garlic clove, minced

10 ounces button or cremini mushrooms, thinly sliced

½ teaspoon kosher salt

½ teaspoon freshly ground black pepper

1 cup pearl barley, rinsed and drained

3 cups reduced-sodium chicken broth

½ cup frozen green peas (thawed)

In a large saucepan, heat the olive oil over medium heat. Add the onion and garlic and cook until the onion is softened, about 3 minutes. Add the mushrooms, salt, and pepper and continue cooking until the mushrooms have softened and released their juice, about 5 minutes. Stir in the barley and cook, stirring, for 1 minute. Add the broth and bring to a boil. Reduce the heat to a simmer, cover, and cook for 35 to 40 minutes, until the broth is absorbed and the barley is soft. Stir in the peas, cover, and let sit for 5 minutes before serving.

NUTRITION PER ½-CUP SERVING

CAL	FAT*	SAT FAT	CHOLEST	SODIUM	CARB	DIET FIBER	SUGARS	PROTEIN
143	4 g	1 g	0 mg	258 mg	23 g	5 g	2 g	5 g

*FAT: 0 g EPA; 0 g DHA; <1 g ALA

From the kitchen of Dr. Janet

CHEF KEITH BLAUSCHILD'S QUINOA
WITH WALNUTS AND CURRANTS

SERVES 6

Rinse the quinoa in a fine-mesh strainer with cool running water before cooking to remove the saponin, a natural coating on the quinoa that can irritate the stomach if not removed. Some quinoa is sold prerinsed.

- 1 cup quinoa, rinsed
- 2 cups reduced-sodium chicken or vegetable broth
- ¼ cup dried currants
- ½ cup chopped walnuts, toasted
- ¼ cup finely sliced scallions, white and green parts (2 thin scallions)

In a saucepan, bring the quinoa and broth to a boil. Add the currants, cover, and reduce the heat to low. Cook for 15 minutes. Turn off the heat, leave covered, and let sit for 5 minutes. After 5 minutes, uncover the pan and lightly fluff the quinoa with a fork to separate the grains. Gently stir in the walnuts and scallions. Serve warm or at room temperature.

NUTRITION PER ½-CUP SERVING

CAL	FAT*	SAT FAT	CHOLEST	SODIUM	CARB	DIET FIBER	SUGARS	PROTEIN
194	8 g	1 g	0 mg	192 mg	26 g	3 g	4 g	7 g

*FAT: 0 g EPA; 0 g DHA; 1 g ALA

From the kitchen of
Parkland Chef Catering
2151 Riverside Drive
Coral Springs, Florida

CHEF JULIE KORHUMEL'S WILD RICE SALAD
SERVES 8

If wild rice isn't available, this salad can be made with 2½ cups of another cooked whole grain, such as brown rice or wheat berries.

    2½ cups cooked wild rice (about 1 cup uncooked)
    ⅔ cup chopped dried figs
    ½ cup chopped flat-leaf parsley
    ⅓ cup chopped red bell pepper
    ¼ cup slivered almonds, toasted
    ¼ cup fresh lemon juice
    2 tablespoons chopped red onion
    2 tablespoons extra virgin olive oil
    ¼ teaspoon kosher salt
    ¼ teaspoon freshly ground black pepper

Toss all of the ingredients together and serve cold.

NUTRITION PER ½-CUP SERVING

CAL	FAT*	SAT FAT	CHOLEST	SODIUM	CARB	DIET FIBER	SUGARS	PROTEIN
138	5 g	1 g	0 mg	40 mg	21 g	3 g	7 g	3 g

*FAT: 0 g EPA; 0 g DHA; <1 g ALA

From the kitchen of
Julie's Gourmet Catering
Libertyville, Illinois

CHEF KEITH BLAUSCHILD'S
BRAISED FRENCH GREEN LENTILS
SERVES 4

Simple on their own or served with Cornmeal-Crusted Salmon (page 323).

1 tablespoon extra virgin olive oil
¼ cup finely chopped onion
¼ cup finely diced carrot
1 garlic clove, minced
2 cups reduced-sodium chicken broth
½ cup green lentils
¼ cup diced sun-dried tomatoes
½ teaspoon kosher salt
Pinch of freshly ground black pepper
1 tablespoon chopped fresh marjoram

In a saucepan, heat the olive oil over medium heat. Add the onion, carrot, and garlic and cook until the garlic is golden. Add the broth, lentils, tomatoes, salt, and pepper. Bring to a simmer, cover, and cook for 1 hour, until the lentils are soft. Remove from the heat and stir in the marjoram. Serve in a shallow bowl as a side dish or with a piece of Cornmeal-Crusted Salmon on top.

NUTRITION PER ⅔-CUP SERVING

CAL	FAT*	SAT FAT	CHOLEST	SODIUM	CARB	DIET FIBER	SUGARS	PROTEIN
137	4 g	1 g	0 mg	426 mg	18 g	8 g	3 g	9 g

*FAT: 0 g EPA; 0 g DHA; <1 g ALA

*From the kitchen of
Parkland Chef Catering
2151 Riverside Drive
Coral Springs, Florida*

CHEF JULIE KORHUMEL'S
CURRIED WHOLE-WHEAT COUSCOUS WITH CHICKPEAS
SERVES 8

Mix the ingredients together and enjoy this healthy, tasty side dish.

- 1 cup whole-wheat couscous
- 2 tablespoons extra virgin olive oil
- 1 tablespoon honey
- ½ teaspoon curry powder
- ¼ teaspoon kosher salt
- Juice of ½ lemon
- ½ cup golden raisins
- ½ cup cooked chickpeas
- 2 tablespoons chopped scallion
- 2 tablespoons finely chopped flat-leaf parsley

In a saucepan, bring 1½ cups water to a boil. Stir in the couscous, cover, reduce the heat to low, and simmer for 5 minutes, until all the water is absorbed. Turn off the heat and let sit for 5 minutes. Meanwhile, in a small bowl, combine the olive oil, honey, curry powder, salt, and lemon juice. After the couscous is cooked, remove the lid and gently stir with a fork to fluff and separate the couscous grains. Gently stir in the raisins, chickpeas, scallion, parsley, and dressing. Serve warm or at room temperature.

NUTRITION PER ½-CUP SERVING

CAL	FAT*	SAT FAT	CHOLEST	SODIUM	CARB	DIET FIBER	SUGARS	PROTEIN
165	5 g	1 g	1 mg	76 mg	28 g	2 g	8 g	4 g

*FAT: 0 g EPA; 0 g DHA; <1 g ALA

From the kitchen of
Julie's Gourmet Catering
Libertyville, Illinois

CHEF KEITH BLAUSCHILD'S KALE WITH WHITE BEANS, GOLDEN RAISINS, AND ORANGE ESSENCE

SERVES 4

Beautiful and simple, these beans are an elegant side dish.

- 1 cup very finely chopped raw kale
- 1 cup canned white beans, drained
- ¼ cup golden raisins
- ½ cup mandarin orange segments, drained
- 1 tablespoon white wine vinegar
- 1 tablespoon extra virgin olive oil
- ½ teaspoon kosher salt
- ½ teaspoon freshly ground black pepper

In a medium bowl, combine all of the ingredients. Refrigerate and serve chilled.

NUTRITION PER ½-CUP SERVING

CAL	FAT*	SAT FAT	CHOLEST	SODIUM	CARB	DIET FIBER	SUGARS	PROTEIN
163	7 g	2 g	3 mg	295 mg	23 g	3 g	8 g	5 g

*FAT: 0 g EPA; 0 g DHA; <1 g ALA

From the kitchen of
Parkland Chef Catering
2151 Riverside Drive
Coral Springs, Florida

CHEF MARIO SPINA'S BRANZINO
WITH BROCCOLI RABE
SERVES 4

Branzino is a popular fish in the Mediterranean area. The secret to delicious branzino—or any fish, for that matter—is to not overcook it. In general, for fully cooked pieces of fish, the rule of thumb is 10 minutes total per inch of thickness of the fillet. If branzino isn't available, substitute red snapper or Chilean sea bass.

¼ cup all-purpose flour
¼ cup extra virgin olive oil
4 garlic cloves, roughly chopped
½ teaspoon crushed red pepper flakes
Four 6-ounce branzino fillets
½ cup dry white wine, such as Chardonnay
One recipe Braised Broccoli Rabe (page 302)
2 teaspoons fresh lemon juice
2 tablespoons fresh oregano
¼ teaspoon kosher salt
¼ teaspoon freshly ground black pepper

Place the flour in a shallow dish. In a large skillet, heat the olive oil over medium heat. Add the garlic and red pepper flakes and cook for 1 minute, but do not brown the garlic. Meanwhile, flour both sides of the fish fillets and place them in the skillet, skin side up. Cook for about 4 minutes. Turn the fish, pour in the wine, cover, and cook for 4 more minutes. Uncover and continue to cook for about 2 more minutes, or until when a fork is twisted in the center of the fillet, the flesh separates easily. Remove the fish to a platter with the Braised Broccoli Rabe. Place the same skillet over medium-high heat. Add the lemon juice, oregano, salt, and pepper. Scrape the pan with a wooden spoon and swirl the pan juices until slightly thickened. Pour the pan sauce over the fish.

NUTRITION PER 6-OUNCE SERVING

CAL	FAT*	SAT FAT	CHOLEST	SODIUM	CARB	DIET FIBER	SUGARS	PROTEIN
432	25 g	4 g	70 mg	231 mg	13 g	4 g	<1 g	37 g

*FAT: <1 g EPA; 1 g DHA; <1 g ALA

From the kitchen of
Mario Ristorante Italiano and Wine Bar
6370 North State Road 7
Coconut Creek, Florida

CHEF MARIO SPINA'S MUSSELS MARINARA

SERVES 4

Fresh mussels served in a garlicky broth makes an exquisite appetizer or entrée.

- 2 pounds Prince Edward mussels
- ¼ cup extra virgin olive oil
- 4 garlic cloves, chopped
- ½ teaspoon crushed red pepper flakes
- ¼ cup dry white wine, such as Chardonnay
- One 16-ounce can no-salt-added whole tomatoes
- 2 tablespoons chopped fresh oregano
- 2 tablespoons chopped fresh parsley

With a stiff brush, wash the mussels in cool running water. Pull off and discard the dark strings attached to the mussel. Throw away any mussels that are not closed or do not close when tapped. In a large skillet with a lid, heat the olive oil over medium heat. Add the garlic and red pepper flakes and cook for several minutes until the garlic is golden. Add the mussels, cover, and cook for 2 minutes. Remove the lid. The mussels should be starting to open. Add the wine, increase the heat to medium high, and cook to slightly thicken the wine, about 5 more minutes. At this point all the mussels should be wide open. Add the tomatoes and their juice, crushing the tomatoes with your hands as you add them. Stir, cover, and cook for 5 minutes. Garnish with the oregano and parsley.

NUTRITION PER 8-OUNCE SERVING

CAL	FAT*	SAT FAT	CHOLEST	SODIUM	CARB	DIET FIBER	SUGARS	PROTEIN
364	19 g	3 g	64 mg	665 mg	15 g	2 g	3 g	28 g

*FAT: 0 g EPA; 0 g DHA; <1 g ALA

From the kitchen of
Mario Ristorante Italiano and Wine Bar
6370 North State Road 7
Coconut Creek, Florida

CHEF MARIO SPINA'S GRILLED SWORDFISH
SERVES 2

Delicious served with a side of Braised Broccoli Rabe (page 302)

Two 6-ounce center-cut swordfish fillets
Juice of 2 lemons
6 tablespoons extra virgin olive oil
2 garlic cloves, chopped
2 tablespoons chopped fresh oregano or mint
½ teaspoon kosher salt
1 teaspoon freshly ground black pepper

Place the fish fillets in a shallow dish. In a small bowl, mix the lemon juice, olive oil, garlic, oregano, salt, and black pepper. Pour half the marinade over the fish and refrigerate for 1 hour. Preheat a grill or sauté pan to medium-high heat. Grill or sauté the fish for about 5 minutes on each side, depending on the thickness and desired degree of doneness. Meanwhile, heat the remaining marinade in a small saucepan or in the skillet used to cook the swordfish, until boiling, and boil for 1 minute. Serve the hot marinade over grilled fish with a pinch of fresh mint for garnish.

NUTRITION PER 6-OUNCE SERVING

CAL	FAT*	SAT FAT	CHOLEST	SODIUM	CARB	DIET FIBER	SUGARS	PROTEIN
395	27 g	5 g	66 mg	294 mg	3 g	<1 g	1 g	34 g

*FAT: <1 g EPA; 1 g DHA; <1 g ALA

From the kitchen of
Mario Ristorante Italiano and Wine Bar
6370 North State Road 7
Coconut Creek, Florida

CHEF KERN MATTEI'S STEAMED RED SNAPPER WITH BLACK BEAN SAUCE

SERVES 2

Black bean sauce is found in most supermarkets in the Asian food section. Any firm whitefish fillet substitutes well for the red snapper. You can also use a whole fish; just make three deep, diagonal gashes on each side of the fish. For steaming, use a traditional Chinese steamer or an electric steamer, or simply make your own stovetop steamer using steamer cookware.

    Two 6-ounce red snapper fillets
    1 tablespoon black bean sauce
    3 garlic cloves, chopped
    1 teaspoon oyster sauce
    ½ teaspoon sugar
    ½ teaspoon dry white wine, such as Chardonnay
    ¼ teaspoon kosher salt
    3 tablespoons extra virgin olive oil
    1 teaspoon red bell pepper, finely chopped
    1 red bell pepper, seeded and cut into thin strips
    2 scallions, one finely chopped and one cut into thin strips
    3 cilantro sprigs

Place the fish on a heatproof plate that fits inside the steamer. In a small bowl, mix the black bean sauce, garlic, oyster sauce, sugar, wine, and salt. Whisk in the olive oil. Add 1 teaspoon finely chopped bell pepper and the finely chopped scallion. Generously brush the sauce on the fish. Place the plate in the steamer and steam over briskly boiling water until the fish turns opaque and flakes easily with a fork, 10 to 12 minutes, depending on the thickness of the fish. Remove the fish to a platter and garnish with the bell pepper strips, sliced scallion, and cilantro.

NUTRITION PER 6-OUNCE SERVING

CAL	FAT*	SAT FAT	CHOLEST	SODIUM	CARB	DIET FIBER	SUGARS	PROTEIN
396	23 g	3 g	63 mg	417 mg	10 g	3 g	5 g	37 g

*FAT: <1 g EPA; <1 g DHA; <1 g ALA

From the kitchen of
Mai-Kai Restaurant
3599 North Federal Highway
Fort Lauderdale, Florida

CHEF KERN MATTEI'S PAN-SEARED SALMON

SERVES 4

A simple preparation for a fresh piece of salmon. Serve with Apple Carrot Salad (page 287)

Four 6-ounce fresh salmon fillets
1 tablespoon reduced-sodium soy sauce
1 tablespoon extra virgin olive oil

Place the salmon fillets in a baking dish. Drizzle the soy sauce over the salmon and let it sit for 15 minutes. In a large skillet, heat the olive oil over medium-high heat. Sear the salmon for 4 to 5 minutes on each side until the fish flakes easily with a fork, depending on the thickness of the fillet.

NUTRITION PER SERVING (6 OUNCES SALMON)

CAL	FAT*	SAT FAT	CHOLEST	SODIUM	CARB	DIET FIBER	SUGARS	PROTEIN
390	22 g	4 g	100 mg	200 mg	0 g	0 g	0 g	35 g

*FAT: 1 g EPA; 2 g DHA; <1 g ALA

From the kitchen of
Mai-Kai Restaurant
3599 North Federal Highway
Fort Lauderdale, Florida

CHEF JULIE KORHUMEL'S STEAMED HALIBUT AND FRESH VEGETABLES IN PARCHMENT PAPER

SERVES 1

Steamed, but full of color from the fresh vegetables.

> One 6-ounce halibut fillet
> 1 tablespoon extra virgin olive oil
> ½ teaspoon Mrs. Dash seasoning
> One ¼-inch-thick slice onion
> ¼ red bell pepper, seeded and thinly sliced
> 7 grape tomatoes, halved
> Four ¼-inch slices zucchini
> 1 tablespoon chopped fresh dill
> ½ teaspoon lemon zest
> 1 tablespoon fresh lemon juice
> Freshly ground black pepper

Preheat the oven to 450° F. Fold a 10-inch square of parchment paper in half on the diagonal to form a triangle and press a crease along the fold. Open the parchment and place on a baking sheet. Lay the fish fillet on the parchment, with one long edge of the fish along the middle of the crease in the paper. Drizzle the fish with the olive oil and season with Mrs. Dash (an alternative salt-free seasoning available in the spice section of your local supermarket). Arrange the onion, bell pepper, tomatoes, and zucchini on top of and around the fish. Sprinkle with the dill, lemon zest, lemon juice, and pepper to taste. Fold the other half of the parchment over the fish. Make several small overlapping folds along the edges and seal with a paper clip. Bake until the paper is puffed, about 12 minutes. To open, use a sharp pair of kitchen shears to cut an X in the top of the fish package, using caution because the steam is very hot.

NUTRITION PER 6-OUNCE SERVING

CAL	FAT*	SAT FAT	CHOLEST	SODIUM	CARB	DIET FIBER	SUGARS	PROTEIN
354	16 g	2 g	81 mg	189 mg	19 g	4 g	9 g	35 g

*FAT: 0 g EPA; 0 g DHA; <1 g ALA

From the kitchen of
Julie's Gourmet Catering
Libertyville, Illinois

CHEF KEITH BLAUSCHILD'S CORNMEAL-CRUSTED SALMON OVER BRAISED LENTILS

SERVES 4

The fresh taste of salmon paired with earthy lentils makes for a hearty meal.

> Four 6-ounce salmon fillets
> ½ cup plus 1 tablespoon orange juice
> 1 teaspoon honey
> 2 tablespoons yellow cornmeal
> ½ teaspoon ground cumin
> ¼ teaspoon granulated garlic
> ¼ teaspoon kosher salt
> ¼ teaspoon freshly ground black pepper
> 2 teaspoons extra virgin olive oil
> One recipe Braised French Green Lentils (page 314)

Place the salmon in a glass baking dish. In a small bowl, mix 1 tablespoon orange juice and the honey. Brush the orange-honey mixture on the salmon. In another small bowl, mix the cornmeal, cumin, garlic, salt, and pepper. Sprinkle evenly over the fish. In a large skillet, heat the olive oil over medium-high heat. Cook the salmon for 2 minutes on each side. Pour in ½ cup orange juice, cover, and cook for 3 minutes. Uncover and let the orange juice reduce until dry, about 3 minutes. The fish should be done at this point, depending on the thickness of the fillet. Spoon the lentils into a shallow bowl and serve the salmon on top of the lentils.

NUTRITION PER SERVING (6 OUNCES SALMON)

CAL	FAT*	SAT FAT	CHOLEST	SODIUM	CARB	DIET FIBER	SUGARS	PROTEIN
460	25 g	5 g	60 mg	560 mg	33 g	3 g	16 g	25 g

*FAT: 1 g EPA; 2 g DHA; <1 g ALA

*From the kitchen of
Parkland Chef Catering
2151 Riverside Drive
Coral Springs, Florida*

CHEF KEITH BLAUSCHILD'S TUNA ROMESCO

SERVES 4

A meaty tuna steak topped with a fresh, spicy, almond-studded tomato sauce.

Four 6-ounce tuna steaks
½ teaspoon kosher salt
½ teaspoon freshly ground black pepper
1 plum tomato, halved and seeded
1 tablespoon extra virgin olive oil
1 teaspoon minced garlic
¼ cup blanched almonds
¼ cup sun-dried tomato
¼ cup chopped roasted red bell pepper
Pinch of crushed red pepper flakes
1 tablespoon red wine vinegar
1 tablespoon chopped fresh parsley
Nonstick cooking spray

Season the tuna with the salt and pepper and refrigerate until ready to cook. Roughly chop the tomato. In a skillet, heat the olive oil over medium heat. Add the garlic and almonds and sauté for several minutes until the garlic turns golden but not too brown. Add the plum tomato, sun-dried tomato, bell pepper, and red pepper flakes. Cook until the tomato is soft. Let cool. Place the tomato mixture in the container of a blender and purée until smooth. Remove to a bowl and stir in the vinegar and parsley. To cook the tuna, spray the fillets lightly with nonstick cooking spray. Heat a nonstick skillet or grill to high heat. Cook for 4 to 5 minutes on each side, depending on thickness and desired degree of doneness.

NUTRITION PER SERVING (6 OUNCES TUNA AND ¼ CUP SAUCE)

CAL	FAT*	SAT FAT	CHOLEST	SODIUM	CARB	DIET FIBER	SUGARS	PROTEIN
285	10 g	1 g	77 mg	307 mg	6 g	2 g	2 g	43 g

*FAT: <1 g EPA; <1 g DHA; <1 g ALA

From the kitchen of
Parkland Chef Catering
2151 Riverside Drive
Coral Springs, Florida

CHEF KEITH BLAUSCHILD'S SHALLOW-POACHED SALMON WITH FENNEL AND SAFFRON

SERVES 4

Some clam juices are high in sodium. Look for brands such as Bar Harbor, Blue Crab Bay, Bookbinder's, and Look's clam juice because they are lower in sodium.

Four 6-ounce salmon fillets
½ teaspoon kosher salt
½ teaspoon freshly ground black pepper
Nonstick cooking spray
1 fennel bulb
1 tablespoon extra virgin olive oil
2 garlic cloves, minced
1 large tomato, seeded and diced
1 cup low-sodium clam juice
½ cup dry white wine, such as Chardonnay
¼ teaspoon saffron

Season the salmon with salt and pepper. In a nonstick skillet sprayed with nonstick cooking spray, brown the salmon on both sides, about 2 minutes. Remove the salmon from the skillet and set aside. Meanwhile, trim the greens off the fennel bulb and reserve for a garnish. Thinly slice the fennel bulb, discarding the inner core. In a large, deep skillet heat the olive oil over medium heat. Add the fennel and cook until tender, about 4 minutes. Add the garlic and lightly brown. Add the tomato, clam juice, wine, and saffron. Bring to a gentle boil and add the salmon fillets. Cover and cook for 8 minutes. Uncover and cook for 1 more minute. Remove the salmon to a shallow bowl and increase the heat to medium-high. Reduce the tomato-fennel broth until thickened, about 5 minutes. Serve the broth over the fish. Garnish with chopped fennel fronds.

NUTRITION PER SERVING (6 OUNCES SALMON AND ABOUT ¾ CUP BROTH)

CAL	FAT*	SAT FAT	CHOLEST	SODIUM	CARB	DIET FIBER	SUGARS	PROTEIN
400	22 g	4 g	100 mg	679 mg	8 g	2 g	1 g	37 g

*FAT: 1 g EPA; 2 g DHA; <1 g ALA

From the kitchen of
Parkland Chef Catering
2151 Riverside Drive
Coral Springs, Florida

CHEF KEITH BLAUSCHILD'S
YELLOWTAIL EN PAPILLOTE

SERVES 4

Marinated fresh vegetables and herbs top the steamed tuna, making for a fresh, light meal. Have ready four 10-inch squares of parchment paper. Heavy-duty foil can be used if parchment is not available.

1 medium zucchini, julienned

1 medium yellow squash, julienned

1 small red bell pepper, seeded and julienned

2 tablespoons extra virgin olive oil

2 tablespoons chopped fresh oregano

2 tablespoons chopped fresh parsley

Juice of 1 lemon

¼ cup dry white wine, such as Chardonnay

Pinch of salt

Freshly ground black pepper

Four 6-ounce yellowtail fillets

Preheat the oven to 375°F. Place the zucchini, yellow squash, and bell pepper in a medium bowl. Toss with the olive oil, oregano, parsley, lemon juice, wine, salt, and pepper. Let sit at room temperature for 15 minutes. Meanwhile, fold each square of parchment paper in half on the diagonal to form a triangle. Open the parchment. Lay one yellowtail fillet on the parchment, lining up the edge of the fillet with the center fold of the paper. Top with one-fourth of the vegetable mix. Fold the other half of the parchment over the fish. Make several small overlapping folds along the edges and seal with a paper clip. Transfer to a baking sheet. Repeat with the remaining parchment, yellowtail, and vegetables. Bake until the paper is puffed, about 22 minutes. To open, use a sharp pair of kitchen shears to cut an X in the top of the fish package, using caution because the steam is very hot.

NUTRITION PER 6-OUNCE SERVING

CAL	FAT*	SAT FAT	CHOLEST	SODIUM	CARB	DIET FIBER	SUGARS	PROTEIN
354	16 g	3 g	94 mg	123 mg	8 g	3 g	4 g	42 g

*FAT: 0 g EPA; 0 g DHA; <1 g ALA

From the kitchen of
Parkland Chef Catering
2151 Riverside Drive
Coral Springs, Florida

CHEF KEITH BLAUSCHILD'S SHRIMP
WITH ARTICHOKE-GARLIC SAUCE

SERVES 4

Full of artichokes, garlic, and fresh herbs, this shrimp dish is a refreshing meal.

2 tablespoons extra virgin olive oil

2 tablespoons chopped shallot

1 tablespoon chopped garlic

½ cup dry sherry

1 pound 16- to 20-count shrimp, peeled and deveined

One 14-ounce can artichoke hearts packed in water, drained
  and roughly chopped

1 cup reduced-sodium chicken broth

1 tablespoon chopped fresh sage

1 tablespoon chopped fresh parsley

¼ teaspoon kosher salt

½ teaspoon freshly ground black pepper

In a large skillet, heat the olive oil over medium heat. Add the shallot and garlic and cook for several minutes until lightly browned. Add the sherry, increase the heat to high, and cook until the sherry reduces, about 2 minutes. Add the shrimp and cook until they turn pink and start to curl, about 1 to 2 minutes. Remove the shrimp from the pan and transfer to a serving bowl. Return the skillet to medium-high heat and add the artichoke hearts and broth, scraping any bits off the bottom of the pan. Cook for about 3 minutes, until the sauce is slightly thickened. Stir in the sage and parsley. Season with the salt and pepper. Pour the sauce over the shrimp and serve.

NUTRITION PER SERVING (5 SHRIMP AND ½ CUP SAUCE)

CAL	FAT*	SAT FAT	CHOLEST	SODIUM	CARB	DIET FIBER	SUGARS	PROTEIN
256	8 g	1 g	53 mg	462 mg	28 g	12 g	2 g	16 g

*FAT: <1 g EPA; <1 g DHA; <1 g ALA

From the kitchen of
Parkland Chef Catering
2151 Riverside Drive
Coral Springs, Florida

DR. JANET'S FLOURLESS DARK CHOCOLATE BROWNIES WITH WALNUTS

SERVES 16

A dark, moist chocolaty treat.

Nonstick cooking spray
One 15-ounce can black beans, drained and rinsed
¾ cup packed Splenda Brown Sugar Blend
½ cup quick-cooking oats
¼ cup unsweetened dark cocoa powder
¼ cup extra virgin olive oil
1 tablespoon espresso powder
2 tablespoons ground flaxseeds
1 teaspoon vanilla extract
¼ teaspoon salt
½ cup chopped walnuts

Preheat the oven to 350°F. Spray a 9-inch baking pan with nonstick cooking spray. Place the black beans in a mixing bowl. Add the brown sugar, oats, cocoa powder, olive oil, espresso powder, flaxseeds, vanilla, and salt. With an electric mixer, blend the ingredients until the black beans are mushed up and the mixture is smooth, about 2 minutes. Scrape the batter into the prepared pan, top with walnuts, and bake for 30 to 35 minutes, until the edges pull away from the sides of the pan and the middle of the brownies is firm. Let cool before slicing into 16 pieces.

NUTRITION PER SERVING (1 BROWNIE)

CAL	FAT*	SAT FAT	CHOLEST	SODIUM	CARB	DIET FIBER	SUGARS	PROTEIN
140	6 g	1 g	1 mg	89 mg	16 g	2 g	<1 g	3 g

*FAT: 0 g EPA; 0 g DHA; 1 g ALA

From the kitchen of Dr. Janet

DR. JANET'S QUICK, HEALTHY
(AND SINFULLY SATISFYING)
DARK HOT CHOCOLATE

SERVES 1

Perfect for a sweet treat on a cold winter's day.

- 2 tablespoons dark unsweetened cocoa powder
- 2 packets Splenda (or sweetener of choice)
- 12 fluid ounces light soy milk
- ⅛ teaspoon vanilla extract
- 2 tablespoons fat-free whipped topping

In a large microwavable mug, mix the cocoa powder with the sweetener. Add the soy milk and vanilla and microwave on high power for 1 minute. Remove from the microwave, stir, and return to the microwave for an additional 90 seconds. Top with whipped topping—feel free to add more as desired.

NUTRITION PER 1-CUP SERVING

CAL	FAT*	SAT FAT	CHOLEST	SODIUM	CARB	DIET FIBER	SUGARS	PROTEIN
154	4 g	1 g	0 mg	186 mg	23 g	5 g	12 g	11 g

*FAT: 0 g EPA; 0 g DHA; 0 g ALA

From the kitchen of Dr. Janet

PREVENT A SECOND HEART ATTACK DAILY CHECKLIST

	MONDAY	TUESDAY	WEDNESDAY
PILLS (as prescribed)			
Prescription medication	___	___	___
statin*	___	___	___
aspirin*			
beta-blocker*	___	___	___
ace inhibitor*	___	___	___
Lovaza fish pill*	___	___	___
optional supplements	___	___	___
plant sterols**	___	___	___
psyllium seed husk**	___	___	___
vitamin D3+	___	___	___
niacin+	___	___	___
FOOD (daily)			
extra virgin olive oil	___ ___	___ ___	___ ___
greens and other vegetables	___ ___ ___	___ ___ ___	___ ___ ___
figs or other fruit	___ ___ ___	___ ___ ___	___ ___ ___
lentils or other legumes	___	___	___
salmon and other fatty fish (3x/week)	___	___	
walnuts and flaxseeds	___ ___	___ ___	___ ___
oatmeal + whole grains	___ ___	___ ___	___ ___
red wine with a meal***	___	___	___
dark chocolate	___	___	___
EXERCISE++			
walking (daily)	___	___	___
strength training (2x/week)	___	___	___

*All prescription medication must be taken under your personal physician's recommendation and supervision.

**These supplements help reduce LDL cholesterol. For recommended dosages please refer to my previous book, *Cholesterol Down: 10 Simple Steps to Lower Your Cholesterol in 4 Weeks—Without Prescription Drugs* (Three Rivers Press, December 2006).

PREVENT A SECOND HEART ATTACK DAILY CHECKLIST

THURSDAY	FRIDAY	SATURDAY	SUNDAY
—	—	—	—
—	—	—	—
—	—	—	—
—	—	—	—
—	—	—	—
—	—	—	—
—	—	—	—
—	—	—	—
—	—	—	—
—	—	—	—

— —	— —	— —	— —
- - - - -	- - - - -	- - - - -	- - - - -
— —	— — —	— —	— — —
—	—	—	—
—	—	—	—
— —	— —	— —	— —
— —	— —	— —	— —
—	—	—	—
—	—	—	—

—	—	—	—
—	—	—	—

+To be taken under your personal physician's recommendation and supervision.

***Drink alcoholic beverages only if you and your personal physician agree that you can drink safely.

++You must receive clearance from your personal physician before you begin this (or any) exercise program.

Notes

Introduction

1. Y. Ma et al., "Dietary quality 1 year after diagnosis of coronary heart disease," *Journal of the American Dietetic Association* (108) 2008: 240–246.

2. American Heart Association, *Heart Disease and Stroke Statistics— 2010 Update* (Dallas, TX: American Heart Association, 2010).

3. J. S. Skinner et al., "Secondary prevention for patients after a myocardial infarction: Summary of NICE guidance," *British Medical Journal* 334 (2007): 1112–1113.

4. M. de Lorgeril et al., "Mediterranean diet, traditional risk factors, and the rate of cardiovascular complications after myocardial infarction: Final report of the Lyon Diet Heart Study," *Circulation* 99 (1999): 779–785.

Chapter 1

1. Nicole Gaskins et al., "Poor nutritional habits: a modifiable predecessor of chronic illness? A North Carolina family medicine research network (NC-FM-RN) study," *Journal of the American Board of Family Medicine* 20 (2007): 124–134.

2. Robert S. Lees, "Prevention of atherosclerosis progression in asymptomatic healthy elderly," *American Journal of Clinical Nutrition* 86 (2007) (suppl.): 1569S–1571S.

3. M. Rodríguez-Morán et al., "Dietary factors related to the increase of cardiovascular risk factors in traditional Tepehuanos communities from Mexico: A 10 year follow-up study," *Nutrition, Metabolism & Cardiovascular Diseases* (2008): doi:10.1016/j.numecd.2008.08.005.

4. Henry C. McGill Jr. and C. Alex McMahan, "Starting earlier to prevent heart disease," *Journal of the American Medical Association* 290 (2003): 2320–2322.

5. William F. Enos, Robert H. Holmes, and James Beyer, "Coronary disease among United States soldiers killed in action in Korea," *Journal of the American Medical Association* 152 (1953): 1090–1093.

6. J. J. McNamara et al., "Coronary artery disease in combat casualties in Vietnam," *Journal of the American Medical Association* 216 (1971): 1185–1187.

7. A. Joseph et al., "Manifestations of coronary atherosclerosis in young trauma victims—an autopsy study," *Journal of the American College of Cardiology* 22, no. 2 (1993): 459–467.

8. Marietta Charakida, Dimitris Tousoulis, and Christodoulos Stefanadis, "Early atherosclerosis in childhood: diagnostic approaches and therapeutic treatment," *International Journal of Cardiology* 109 (2006): 152–159.

9. Gerald Berenson et al., "Association between multiple cardiovascular risk factors and atherosclerosis in children and young adults," *New England Journal of Medicine* 388 (1998): 1650–1656.

10. Jack P. Strong et al., "Prevalence of atherosclerosis in adolescents and young adults: Implications for prevention from the Pathobiological Determinants of Atherosclerosis in Youth study," *Journal of the American Medical Association* 281, no. 8 (1999): 727–735.

11. Arcangelo Iannuzzi et al., "Increased carotid intima-media thickness and stiffness in obese children," *Diabetes Care* 27 (2004): 2506–2508.

12. Pam Belluck, "Child obesity seen as warning of heart disease," *New York Times,* November 12, 2008.

13. Jenifer L. Baker, Lina W. Olsen, and Thorkild I. A. Sørensen, "Childhood body-mass index and the risk of coronary heart disease in adulthood," *New England Journal of Medicine* 357 (2007): 2329–2337.

14. Morteza Naghavi et al., "From vulnerable plaque to vulnerable pa-

tient: A call for new definitions and risk assessment strategies: Part I," *Circulation* 108 (2003): 1664–1672.

15. Sidney C. Smith Jr. et al., "AHA/ACC guidelines for secondary prevention for patients with coronary and other atherosclerotic vascular disease: 2006 update: Endorsed by the National Heart, Lung, and Blood Institute," *Circulation* 113 (2006): 2363–2372.

16. Ira Tabas, Kevin Jon Williams, and Jan Borén, "Subendothelial lipoprotein retention as the initiating process in atherosclerosis: Update and therapeutic implications," *Circulation* 116 (2007): 1832–1844.

17. Smith et al., "AHA/ACC guidelines for secondary prevention."

18. Inder M. Singh, Medhi H. Shishehbor, and Benjamin J. Ansell, "High-density lipoprotein as a therapeutic target," *Journal of the American Medical Association* 298, no. 7 (2007): 786–798.

Chapter 2

1. Gregg C. Fonarow, "The global burden of cardiovascular disease," *Nature Clinical Practice Cardiovascular Medicine* 4, no. 10 (2007): 530–531.

2. Valentin Fuster, "Mechanisms leading to myocardial infarction: Insights from studies of vascular biology," *Circulation* 90, no. 4 (1994): 2126–2146.

3. Matthias Barton, Roberta Minotti, and Elvira Haas, "Inflammation and atherosclerosis," *Circulation Research* 101 (2007): 750–751.

4. Steven P. Gieseg et al., "Potential to inhibit growth of atherosclerotic plaque development through modulation of macrophage neopterin/ 7,8-dihydroneopterin synthesis," *British Journal of Pharmacology* 153 (2008): 627–635.

5. Søren Dalager et al., "Artery-related differences in atherosclerosis expression: Implications for atherogenesis and dynamics in intima-media thickness," *Stroke* 38 (2007): 2698–2705; and Russell Ross, "Atherosclerosis—an inflammatory disease," *New England Journal of Medicine* 340, no. 2 (1999): 115–126.

6. Göran K. Hansson, "Inflammation, atherosclerosis, and coronary artery disease," *New England Journal of Medicine* 352 (2005): 1685–1695.

7. Ibid.

8. Henry C. McGill Jr. et al., for the Pathobiological Determinants of Atherosclerosis in Youth (PDAY) research group, "Origin of atherosclerosis in childhood and adolescence," *American Journal of Clinical Nutrition* 72 (2000) (suppl.): 1307S–1315S.

9. Peter Libby, Paul M. Ridker, and Attilio Maseri, "Inflammation and atherosclerosis," *Circulation* 105, no. 9 (March 2002): 1135–1143; and John R. Guyton, "Atherosclerosis—a story of cells, cholesterol, and clots," National Lipid Association, http://www.lipid.org/clinical/patients/1000005.php.

10. Guyton, "Atherosclerosis."

11. Peter Libby, "Inflammation in atherosclerosis," *Nature* 420 (December 2002): 868–874.

12. Guyton, "Atherosclerosis."

13. Valentin Fuster, "Mechanisms leading to myocardial infarction: Insights from studies of vascular biology," *Circulation* 90, no. 4 (1994): 2126–2146.

14. Prediman K. Shah, "Pathophysiology of coronary thrombosis: Role of plaque rupture and plaque erosion," *Progress in Cardiovascular Diseases* 44, no. 5 (2002): 357–368.

15. Dalager et al., "Artery-related differences in atherosclerosis expression."

16. Shah, "Pathophysiology of coronary thrombosis."

17. Christopher K. Glass and Joseph L. Witztum, "Atherosclerosis: The road ahead," *Cell* 104 (2001): 503–516.

Chapter 3

1. D. S. McLaren, "The kingdom of the Keyses," *Nutrition* 13, no. 3 (1997): 249, 253.

2. Ancel Keys, ed., "Coronary heart disease in seven countries," *Circulation* 41 (1970) (suppl. 1): 1–211.

3. Ancel Keys and Margaret Keys, *How to Eat Well and Stay Well the Mediterranean Way* (New York: Doubleday, 1975).

4. P. Leren, "The Oslo diet-heart study: Eleven-year report," *Circulation* 42 (1970): 935–942; J. M. Woodhill et al., "Low fat, low cholesterol diet in secondary prevention of coronary heart disease," *Advances in Experimental and Medical Biology* 109 (1978): 317–331; and Research Committee to the Medical Research Council, "Controlled trial of soya-bean oil in myocardial infarction," *Lancet* 2 (1968): 693–700.

5. Research Committee to the Medical Research Council, "Controlled trial of soya-bean oil."

6. Woodhill et al., "Low fat, low cholesterol diet."

7. Leren, "The Oslo diet-heart study."

8. A. Chait et al., "Rationale of the diet-heart statement of the American Heart Association," Report of the Nutrition Committee, *Circulation* 88 (1993): 3008–3029.

9. M. L. Burr et al., "Effects of changes in fat, fish and fibre intakes on death and myocardial reinfarction: Diet and reinfarction trial (DART)," *Lancet* 334 (1989): 757–761.

10. Michel de Lorgeril et al., "Mediterranean alpha-linolenic acid-rich diet in secondary prevention of coronary heart disease," *Lancet* 343 (1994): 1454–1459.

11. F. Barzi et al., on behalf of GISSI-Prevenzione investigators, "Mediterranean diet and all-causes mortality after myocardial infarction: Results from the GISSI-Prevenzione trial," *European Journal of Clinical Nutrition* 57 (2003): 604–611.

12. R. B. Singh et al., "Randomised controlled trial of cardioprotective diet in patients with acute myocardial infarction: Results of one year follow-up," *British Medical Journal* 304 (1992): 1015–1019.

13. R. B. Singh et al., "Effect of an Indo-Mediterranean diet on progression of coronary artery disease in high risk patients [Indo-Mediterranean diet heart Study]: A randomized single-blind trial," *Lancet* 360 (2002): 1455–1461.

14. R. Estruch et al., "Effects of a Mediterranean-style diet on cardiovascular risk factors: A randomized trial," *Annals of Internal Medicine* 144 (2006): 1–11.

Chapter 4

1. Ancel Keys et al., "The diet and 15-year death rate in the Seven Countries Study," *American Journal of Epidemiology* (1986) 124 (1986): 903–915.

2. Daan Kromhout et al., "Dietary saturated and *trans* fatty acids and cholesterol and 25-year mortality from coronary heart disease: The Seven Countries Study," *American Journal of Preventive Medicine* 24, no. 3 (1995): 308–315.

3. Keith G. Mansfield et al., "A diet high in saturated fat and cholesterol accelerates Simian Immunodeficiency Virus disease progression," *Journal of Infectious Diseases* 196 (2007): 1202–1210.

4. Vikkie A. Mustad et al., "Reducing saturated fat intake is associated with increased levels of LDL receptors on mononuclear cells in healthy men and women," *Journal of Lipid Research* 38 (1997): 459–468.

5. Stephen J. Nicholls et al., "Consumption of saturated fat impairs the anti-inflammatory properties of high-density lipoproteins and endothelial function," *Journal of the American College of Cardiology* 48, no. 4 (2006): 715–720.

6. Frans Kok and Daan Kromhout, "Atherosclerosis—epidemiological studies on the health effects of a Mediterranean diet," *European Journal of Nutrition* 43 (March 2004) (suppl. 1): I/2–5.

7. Food and Nutrition Board, Institute of Medicine of the National Academies, *Dietary Reference Intakes for Energy, Carbohydrate, Fiber, Fat, Fatty Acids, Cholesterol, Protein, and Amino Acids* (Washington, DC: National Academies Press, 2005), http://www.nap.edu.

8. Third Report of the National Cholesterol Education Program (NCEP) Expert Panel on Detection, Evaluation, and Treatment of High Blood Cholesterol in Adults (Adult Treatment Panel III), Final Report, *National Cholesterol Education Program, National Heart, Lung, and Blood Institute, National Institutes of Health, NIH Publication No. 02–5215,* September 2002.

9. Jean-François Mauger et al., "Effect of different forms of dietary hydrogenated fats on LDL particle size," *American Journal of Clinical Nutrition* 78 (2003): 370–375.

10. Dariush Mozaffarian et al., "Trans fatty acids and cardiovascular disease," *New England Journal of Medicine* 345 (2006):1601–1603; and

Qi Sun et al., "A prospective study of trans fatty acids in erythrocytes and risk of coronary heart disease," *Circulation* 115 (2007): 1858–1865.

11. "Food labeling; *trans* fatty acids in nutrition labeling; consumer research to consider nutrient content and health claims and possible footnote or disclosure statements; final rule and proposed rule," *Federal Register* 68, no. 133 (July 11, 2003).

12. Center for Science in the Public Interest, "Trans fat: On the way out," http://www.cspinet.org/transfat.

13. Food and Nutrition Board, *Dietary Reference Intakes for Energy, Carbohydrate, Fiber, Fat, Fatty Acids, Cholesterol, Protein, and Amino Acids.*

14. Robert Kleeman et al., "Atherosclerosis and liver inflammation induced by increased dietary cholesterol intake: A combined transcriptomics and metabolomics analysis," *Genome Biology* 8, no. 9 (2007): R200.1–R200.15.

15. Third Report of the National Cholesterol Education Program (NCEP) Expert Panel, *National Cholesterol Education Program.*

16. Judy Putnam and Shirley Gerrior, "Trends in the U.S. food supply, 1970–97," in *America's Eating Habits: Changes and Consequences* (Washington, DC: USDA Economic Research Service, 1999), 133–160.

17. Daan Kromhout, "On the waves of the Seven Countries Study: A public health perspective on cholesterol," *European Heart Journal* 20 (1999): 796–802.

Chapter 5

1. James Ferro-Luzzi, W. P. T. James, and A. Kafatos, "The high-fat Greek diet: A recipe for all?" *European Journal of Clinical Nutrition* 56 (2002): 796–809.

2. Ancel Keys, ed., "Coronary heart disease in seven countries," *Circulation* 41 (1970) (suppl. 1): 1–211.

3. David Grigg, "Food consumption in the Mediterranean region," *Tijdschrift voor Economische en Sociale Geografie* 90, no. 4 (1999): 391–409.

4. L. I. Serra-Majem et al., "Olive oil and the Mediterranean diet:

Beyond the rhetoric," *European Journal of Clinical Nutrition* 57 (2003) (suppl. 1): S2–S7.

5. Antonia Trichopoulou, "Traditional Mediterranean diet and longevity in the elderly: A review," *Public Health Nutrition* 7, no. 7 (2004): 943–947.

6. Paola Bogani et al., "Postprandial anti-inflammatory and antioxidant effects of extra virgin olive oil," *Atherosclerosis* 190 (2007): 181–186.

7. María-Isabel Covas et al., "The effect of polyphenols in olive oil on heart disease risk factors," *Annals of Internal Medicine* 145 (2006): 333–341.

8. Angelo Azzi et al., "Vitamin E: A sensor and an information transducer of the cell oxidation state," *American Journal of Clinical Nutrition* 62 (1995) (suppl.): 1337S–1346S; and Jan Regnström et al., "Inverse relation between the concentration of low-density-lipoprotein vitamin E and severity of coronary artery disease," *American Journal of Clinical Nutrition* 63 (1996): 377–385.

9. Food and Drug Administration, "FDA allows qualified health claim to decrease risk of coronary heart disease," news release, P04–100, November 1, 2004, http://www.fda.gov/NewsEvents/Newsroom/PressAnnouncements/2004/ucm108368.htm.

10. Bogani et al., "Postprandial anti-inflammatory and antioxidant effects."

11. María-Isabel Covas, "Olive oil and the cardiovascular system," *Pharmacological Research* 55 (2007): 175–186.

12. Francesco Visioli, Giorgio Bellomo, and Claudio Galli, "Free radical-scavenging properties of olive oil polyphenols," *Biochemical and Biophysical Research Communications* 247 (1998): 60–64.

13. Gary K. Beauchamp et al., "Phytochemistry: Ibuprofen-like activity in extra-virgin olive oil," *Nature* 437 (2005): 45–46.

14. S. Terés et al., "Oleic acid content is responsible for the reduction in blood pressure induced by olive oil," *Proceedings of the National Academy of Sciences* 105, no. 37 (2008): 13811–13816.

15. Francisco Pérez-Jiménez, José López-Miranda, and Pedro Mata, "Protective effect of dietary monounsaturated fat on arteriosclerosis: Beyond cholesterol," *Arteriosclerosis* 163 (2002): 385–398.

16. Ibid.

17. Visioli et al., "Free radical-scavenging properties."

18. Anna Petroni et al., "Inhibition of platelet aggregation and eicosanoid production by phenolic components of olive oil," *Thrombosis Research* 78, no. 2 (1995): 151–160.

19. E. Gimeno et al., "Effect of ingestion of virgin olive oil on human low-density lipoprotein composition," *European Journal of Clinical Nutrition* 56 (2002): 114–120.

Chapter 6

1. Ancel Keys, "Diet and public health: Personal reflections," *American Journal of Clinical Nutrition* 61 (1995) (suppl.): 1321S–1323S.

2. Zora Djuric et al., "Design of a Mediterranean exchange list diet implemented by telephone counseling," *Journal of the American Dietetic Association* 108, no. 12 (2008): 2059–2065.

3. Riu Hai Liu, "Health benefits of fruit and vegetables are from additive and synergistic combinations of phytochemicals," *American Journal of Clinical Nutrition* 78 (2003) (suppl.): 517S–520S.

4. Ibid.

5. Joe A. Vinson et al., "Plant flavonoids, especially tea flavonols, are powerful antioxidants using in vitro oxidation model for heart disease," *Journal of Agricultural Food Chemistry* 43 (1995): 2800–2802.

6. Guohua Cao et al., "Serum antioxidant capacity is increased by consumption of strawberries, spinach, red wine or vitamin C in elderly women," *Journal of Nutrition* 128 (1998): 2383–2390.

7. Alexander G. Schauss et al., "Antioxidant capacity and other bioactivities of the freeze-dried Amazonian palm berry, *Euterpe oleraceae mart.* (acai)," *Journal of Agricultural and Food Chemistry* 54 (2006): 8604–8610.

8. Xianli Wu et al., "Development of a database for total antioxidant capacity in foods: A preliminary study," *Journal of Food Composition and Analysis* 17 (2004): 407–422.

9. Winston J. Craig, "Health-promoting properties of common herbs," *American Journal of Clinical Nutrition* 70 (1999) (suppl.): 491S–499S.

10. Adrianne Bendich, "From 1989 to 2001: What have we learned about the 'biological actions of beta-carotene'?" *Journal of Nutrition* 134 (2004): 225S–230S.

11. Alan Mortensen, "Scavenging of benzylperoxyl radicals by carotenoids," *Free Radical Research* 36, no. 2 (2002): 211–216.

12. Chris I. R. Gill et al., "Watercress supplementation in diet reduces lymphocyte DNA damage and alters blood antioxidant status in healthy adults," *American Journal of Clinical Nutrition* 85 (2007): 504–510.

13. Mingzhan Xue et al., "Activation of NF-E2-related factor-2 reverses biochemical dysfunction of endothelial cells induced by hyperglycemia linked to vascular disease," *Diabetes* 57 (2008): 2809–2817.

14. Subramaniam Pennathur and Jay W. Heinecke, "Mechanisms for oxidative stress in diabetic cardiovascular disease," *Antioxidants & Redox Signaling* 9 (2007): 955–969.

15. Craig, "Health-promoting properties of common herbs."

16. L. Tesoriere et al., "Bioactive compounds of caper from Sicily and antioxidant effects in a red meat stimulated gastric digestion," *Journal of Agricultural and Food Chemistry* 55, no. 21 (2007): 8465–8471.

17. Luc Dauchet et al., "Fruit and vegetable consumption and risk of coronary heart disease: A meta-analysis of cohort studies," *Journal of Nutrition* 136 (2006): 2588–2593.

Chapter 7

1. Joe A. Vinson et al., "Dried fruits: Excellent in vitro and in vivo antioxidants," *Journal of the American College of Nutrition* 24, no. 1 (2005): 44–50.

2. Simin Liu et al., "Fruit and vegetable intake and risk of cardiovascular disease: The Women's Health Study," *American Journal of Clinical Nutrition* 72 (2000): 922–928.

3. Q. Su et al., "Identification and quantification of major carotenoids in selected components of the Mediterranean diet: Green leafy vegetables, figs and olive oil," *European Journal of Clinical Nutrition* 56 (2002): 1149–1154.

4. Vinson et al., "Dried fruits."

5. M. A. Martínez-González et al., "Role of fibre and fruit in the Mediterranean diet to protect against myocardial infarction: A case-control study in Spain," *European Journal of Clinical Nutrition* 56 (2002): 715–722.

6. Mary B. Engler and Marguerite M. Engler, "The emerging role of flavonoid-rich cocoa and chocolate in cardiovascular health and disease," *Nutrition Reviews* 64, no. 3 (2006): 109–118.

7. John W. Erdman et al., "Flavonoids and heart health: Proceedings of the ILSI North American flavonoids workshop," *Journal of Nutrition* 137 (2007): 718S–737S.

8. Joe A. Vinson et al., "Phenol antioxidant quantity and quality in foods: Fruits," *Journal of Agricultural and Food Chemistry* 49 (2001): 5315–5321.

9. Claudine Manach et al., "Polyphenols: Food sources and bioavailability," *American Journal of Clinical Nutrition* 79 (2004): 727–747.

10. Michael G. L. Hertog et al., "Dietary antioxidant flavonoids and risk of coronary heart disease," *Lancet* 342 (1993): 1007–1011.

11. Ingrid Ellingsen et al., "Vitamin C consumption is associated with less progression in carotid intima media thickness in elderly men: A 3-year intervention study," *Nutrition, Metabolism & Cardiovascular Diseases* 19 (2009): 8–14.

12. Kristiina Nyyssönen et al., "Vitamin C deficiency and risk of myocardial infarction: Prospective population study of men from eastern Finland," *British Medical Journal* 314 (1997): 2634–2638.

13. Vinson et al., "Dried fruits."

14. Winston J. Craig, "Health-promoting properties of common herbs," *American Journal of Clinical Nutrition* 70 (1999) (suppl.): 491S–499S.

15. Laura Bravo, "Polyphenols: Chemistry, dietary sources, metabolism, and nutritional significance," *Nutrition Reviews* 56, no. 11 (1998): 317–333.

16. Tosca L. Zern and Maria Luz Fernandez, "Cardioprotective effects of dietary polyphenols," *Journal of Nutrition* 135 (2005): 2291–2294.

17. Gudrun Reiterer, Michal Toborek, and Bernhard Hennig, "Quercetin

protects against linoleic acid–induced porcine endothelial cell dysfunction," *Journal of Nutrition* 134 (2004): 771–775.

18. Angel Cogolludo et al., "The dietary flavonoid quercetin activates BKCa currents in coronary arteries via production of H_2O_2. Role in vasodilatation," *Cardiovascular Research* 73, no. 2 (2007): 424–431.

19. Adnan K. Chhatriwalla et al., "Low levels of low-density lipoprotein cholesterol and blood pressure and progression of coronary atherosclerosis," *Journal of the American College of Cardiology* 53 (2009): 1110–1115.

20. Ibid.

21. David W. Harsha et al., "Dietary approaches to stop hypertension: A summary of study results," *Journal of the American Dietetic Association* 99 (1999) (suppl.): S35–S39.

22. Daniela Saes Sartorelli, Laércio Joel Franco, and Marly Augusto Cardosa, "High intake of fruits and vegetables predicts weight loss in Brazilian overweight adults," *Nutrition Research* 28 (2008): 233–238.

23. Liu et al., "Fruit and vegetable intake."

Chapter 8

1. Mercedes Martínez San Ireneo et al., "Clinical features of legume allergy in children from a Mediterranean area," *Annals of Allergy, Asthma, and Immunology* 101 (2008): 179–184.

2. Reay Tannahill, *Food in History* (New York: Crown 1988), 30.

3. Irene Darmadi-Blackberry et al., "Legumes: The most important predictor of survival in older people of different ethnicities," *Asia Pacific Journal of Clinical Nutrition* 13, no. 2 (2004): 217–220.

4. Uriel S. Barzel and Linda K. Massey, "Excess dietary protein can adversely affect bone," *Journal of Nutrition* 128, no. 6 (June 1998): 1051–1053.

5. Susan A. Lanham-New, "The balance of bone health: Tipping the scales in favor of potassium-rich, bicarbonate-rich foods," *Journal of Nutrition* 138 (2008): 172S–177S.

6. Christy Krieg, "The role of diet in the prevention of common kidney stones," *Urologic Nursing* 25, no. 6 (2005): 451–456.

7. Bradley J. Maroni and William E. Mitch, "Role of nutrition in prevention of the progression of renal disease," *Annual Review of Nutrition* 17 (1997): 435–455.

8. C. Spanou et al., "Asssessment of antioxidant activity of extracts from unique Greek varieties of *Leguminosae* plants using *in vitro* assays," *Anticancer Research* 27, 5A (2007): 3403–3410.

9. James W. Anderson and Amy W. Major, "Pulses and lipaemia, short- and long-term effect: Potential in the prevention of cardiovascular disease," *British Journal of Nutrition* 88 (2002) (suppl. 3): S263–S271.

10. American Heart Association, "What is homocysteine?" http://www.americanheart.org/presenter.jhtml?identifier=535.

11. Scott M. Grundy et al., "Diagnosis and management of the metabolic syndrome: An American Heart Association/National Heart, Lung, and Blood Institute scientific statement," *Circulation* 112 (2005): 2735–2752.

12. Jane K. Pittaway, Iain K. Robertson, and Madeleine J. Ball, "Chickpeas may influence fatty acid and fiber intake in an ad libitum diet, leading to small improvements in serum lipid profile and glycemic control," *Journal of the American Dietetic Association* 108, no. 6 (June 2008): 1009–1013.

13. Raquel Villegas et al., "Legume and soy food intake and the incidence of type 2 diabetes in the Shanghai Women's Health Study," *American Journal of Clinical Nutrition* 87, no. 1 (2008): 162–167.

14. Yap-Hang Chan et al., "Isoflavone intake in persons at high risk of cardiovascular events: Implications for vascular endothelial function and the carotid atherosclerotic burden," *American Journal of Clinical Nutrition* 86 (2007): 938–945.

Chapter 9

1. H. O. Bang et al., "The composition of the Eskimo food in northwestern Greenland," *American Journal of Clinical Nutrition* 33 (1980): 2657–2661.

2. Peter Bjerregaard, Gert Mulvad, and Henning Sloth Pedersen, "Cardiovascular risk factors in Inuit of Greenland," *International Journal of Epidemiology* 26, no. 6 (1999): 1182–1190.

3. Clemens von Schacky et al., "The effect of dietary omega-3 fatty acids on coronary atherosclerosis: A randomized, double-blind, placebo-controlled trial," *Annals of Internal Medicine* 130 (1999): 554–562; Sudheera S. D. Nair et al., "Prevention of cardiac arrhythmia by dietary (ω-3) polyunsaturated fatty acids and their mechanism of action," *Journal of Nutrition* 127 (1997): 383–393; and Bang et al., "The composition of the Eskimo food in northwestern Greenland."

4. Ioanna Gouni-Berthold, Wilhelm Krone, and Heiner K. Berthold, "Vitamin D and cardiovascular disease," *Current Vascular Pharmacology* 7, no. 3 (2009): 414–422.

5. Thomas J. Wang et al., "Vitamin D deficiency and risk of cardiovascular disease," *Circulation* 117 (2008): 503–511.

6. Frank B. Hu et al., "Fish and omega-3 fatty acid intake and risk of coronary heart disease in women," *Journal of the American Medical Association* 287 (2002): 1815–1821.

7. John H. Lee et al., "Omega-3 fatty acids for cardioprotection," *Mayo Clinic Proceedings* 83, no. 3 (2008): 324–332.

8. M. L. Burr et al., "Effects of changes in fat, fish and fibre intakes on death and myocardial reinfarction: Diet and Reinfarction Trial (DART)," *Lancet* 334 (1989): 757–761.

9. Carl J. Lavie et al., "Omega-3 polyunsaturated fatty acids and cardiovascular diseases," *Journal of the American College of Cardiology* 54 (2009): 585–594.

10. American Heart Association, "Fish and omega-3 fatty acids," http://www.americanheart.org/presenter.jhtml?identifier=4632.

11. Mitsuhiro Yokoyama, M.D., Ph.D., Kobe University School of Medicine, Kobe, Japan, "Study: Effects of eicosapentaenoic acid (EPA) on major cardiovascular events in hypercholesterolemic patients: The Japan EPA Lipid Intervention Study (JELIS)," in Abhinav Goyal et al., "Highlights from the American Heart Association Scientific Sessions, November 13 to 16, 2005, Dallas, TX," *American Heart Journal* 151, no. 2 (2006): 295–307.

12. American Heart Association, "Fish and omega-3 fatty acids."

13. William S. Harris, "Expert opinion: Omega-3 fatty acids and

bleeding—cause for concern?" *American Journal of Cardiology* 19, no. 99 (6A) (2007): 44C–46C.

14. Lee et al., "Omega-3 fatty acids for cardioprotection."

15. Jordana K. Schmier et al., "The cost-effectiveness of omega-3 supplements for prevention of secondary coronary events," *Managed Care* (2006): 43–50.

16. Lee et al., "Omega-3 fatty acids for cardioprotection."

17. Frank Thies et al., "Association of ω-3 polyunsaturated fatty acids with stability of atherosclerotic plaques: A randomized controlled trial," *Lancet* 361 (2003): 477–485.

18. Nair et al., "Prevention of cardiac arrhythmia."

19. "American Heart Association, "Sudden cardiac death," http://www.americanheart.org/presenter.jhtml?identifier=4741.

20. Michael Miller et al., "Impact of triglyceride levels beyond low-density lipoprotein cholesterol after acute coronary syndrome in the PROVE IT-TIMI 22 trial," *Journal of the American College of Cardiology* 51 (2008): 724–730.

21. American Heart Association, "Fish and omega-3 fatty acids."

22. Trevor A. Mori and Lawrence J. Beilin, "Omega-3 fatty acids and inflammation," *Current Atherosclerosis Reports* 6 (2004): 461–467.

23. Ibid.

24. Bang et al., "The composition of the Eskimo food in northwestern Greenland."

25. Anna L. Choi et al., "Methylmercury exposure and adverse cardiovascular effects in Faroese whaling men," *Environmental Health Perspectives* 117, no. 3 (2009): 367–372.

26. Environmental Protection Agency, "What you need to know about mercury in fish," http://www.epa.gov/waterscience/fish/advice/.

27. Dariush Mozaffarian and Eric B. Rimm, "Fish intake, contaminants, and human health: Evaluating the risks and the benefits," *Journal of the American Medical Association* 296, no. 15 (2006): 1885–1899.

28. Lee et al., "Omega-3 fatty acids for cardioprotection."

Chapter 10

1. Kalish Prasad, "Reduction of serum cholesterol and hypercholesterolemic atherosclerosis in rabbits by secoisolariciresinol diglucoside isolated from flaxseed," *Circulation* 99 (1999): 1355–1362.

2. Artemis P. Simopoulos,"The importance of the ratio of omega-6/omega-3 essential fatty acids," *Biomedicine & Pharmacotherapy* 56, no. 8 (2002): 365–379.

3. Emilio Ros et al., "A walnut diet improves endothelial function in hypercholesterolemic subjects," *Circulation* 109 (2004): 1609–1614.

4. Sujatha Rajaram et al., "Walnuts and fatty fish influence different serum lipid fractions in normal to mildly hyperlipidemic individuals: A randomized controlled study," *American Journal of Clinical Nutrition* 89, no. 5 (2009): 1657S–1663S.

5. Anagha Patade et al., "Flaxseed reduces total and LDL cholesterol concentrations in Native American postmenopausal women," *Journal of Women's Health* 17, no. 3 (2008): 355–366.

6. Margaret A. Allman, M. M. Pena, and D. Pang, "Supplementation with flaxseed oil versus sunflower seed oil in healthy young men consuming a low fat diet: Effects on platelet composition and function," *European Journal of Clinical Nutrition* 49 (1995): 169–178.

7. M. A. Micallef, I. A. Munro, and M. L. Garg, "An inverse relationship between plasma ω-3 fatty acids and C-reactive protein in healthy individuals," *European Journal of Clinical Nutrition* 63 (2009): 1154–1156.

8. Loukianos S. Rallidis et al., "Dietary α-linolenic acid decreases C-reactive protein, serum amyloid A and interleukin-6 in dyslipidaemic patients," *Atherosclerosis* 167 (2003): 237–242.

Chapter 11

1. I. Flight and P. Clifton, "Cereal grains and legumes in the prevention of coronary heart disease and stroke: A review of the literature," *European Journal of Clinical Nutrition* 60 (2006): 1145–1159.

2. Philip B. Mellen et al., "Whole grain intake and cardiovascular disease: A meta-analysis," *Nutrition, Metabolism & Cardiovascular Diseases* 18 (2008): 283–290.

3. Arja T. Erkkilä et al., "Cereal fiber and whole-grain intake are associated with reduced progression of coronary-artery atherosclerosis in postmenopausal women with coronary artery disease," *American Heart Journal* 150 (2005): 94–101.

4. Lin Nie et al., "Avenanthramide, a polphenol from oats, inhibits vascular smooth muscle cell proliferation and enhances nitric oxide," *Atherosclerosis* 186 (2006): 260–266.

5. Judith Hallfrisch and Kay M. Behall, "Mechanisms of the effects of grains on insulin and glucose responses," *Journal of the American College of Nutrition* 19, no. 3 (2000): 320S–325S.

6. Mark A. Pereira et al., "Dietary fiber and risk of coronary heart disease: A pooled analysis of cohort studies," *Archives of Internal Medicine* 164 (2004): 370–376.

7. Institute of Medicine, "Dietary reference intakes for energy, carbohydrate, fiber, fat, fatty acids, cholesterol, protein, and amino acids." http://www.iom.edu/Object.File/Master/4/154/MACRO8pg FINAL.pdf.

8. International Food Information Council Foundation, "Whole grains fact sheet," http://www.ific.org/publications/factsheets/ wholegrainsfs.cfm.

9. Joanne L. Slavin et al., "Plausible mechanisms for the protectiveness of whole grains," *American Journal of Clinical Nutrition* 70 (1999): 459S–463S.

10. U.S. Department of Health and Human Services, "FDA health claim notification for whole-grain foods," http://www.fda.gov/Food/ LabelingNutrition/LabelClaims/FDAModernizationActFDAMA Claims/ucm073639.htm.

11. Harold E. Miller et al., "Antioxidant content of whole-grain breakfast cereals, fruits and vegetables," *Journal of the American College of Nutrition* 19 (2000): 312S–319S.

12. Claudine Manach et al., "Polyphenols: Food sources and bioavailability," *American Journal of Clinical Nutrition* 79, no. 5 (2004): 727–747.

13. Ripple Talati et al., "The effects of barley-derived soluble fiber on serum lipids," *Annals of Family Medicine* 7 (2009): 157–163.

14. Alan J. Flint et al., "Whole grains and incident hypertension in men," *American Journal of Clinical Nutrition* 90 (2009): 493–498.

15. Kay M. Behall et al., "Whole-grain diets reduce blood pressure in mildly hypercholesterolemic men and women," *Journal of the American Dietetic Association* 106 (2006): 1445–1449.

16. Nadine R. Sahyoun et al., "Whole-grain intake is inversely associated with the metabolic syndrome and mortality in older adults," *American Journal of Clinical Nutrition* 83 (2006): 124–131.

17. Hallfrisch and Behall, "Mechanisms of the effects of grains on insulin and glucose responses."

18. Nicola M. McKeown et al., "Whole-grain intake is favorably associated with metabolic risk factors for type 2 diabetes and cardiovascular disease in the Framingham Offspring Study," *American Journal of Clinical Nutrition* 76 (2002): 390–398.

19. Jeroen S. L. de Munter et al., "Whole-grain, bran, and germ intake and risk of type 2 diabetes: A prospective cohort study and systematic review," *PLoS Medicine* 4, no. 8 (2007): 1385–1395.

20. Pauline Koh-Banerjee et al., "Changes in whole-grain, bran, and cereal fiber consumption in relation to 8-y weight gain among men," *American Journal of Clinical Nutrition* 80 (2004): 1237–1245.

Chapter 12

1. Mark Berkowitz, "World's earliest wine," *Archeology* 49, no. 5 (September/October 1996), http://www.archaeology.org/9609/newsbriefs/wine.html.

2. James O'Keefe, Kevin A. Bybee, and Carl J. Lavie, "Alcohol and cardiovascular health: The razor-sharp double-edged sword," *Journal of the American College of Cardiology* 50 (2007): 1009–1014; and Luc Djoussé et al., "Alcohol consumption and risk of cardiovascular disease and death in women: Potential mediating mechanisms," *Circulation* 120 (2009): 237–244.

3. Karen A. Cooper, Mridula Chopra, and David I. Thurnham, "Wine polyphenols and promotion of cardiac health," *Nutrition Research Reviews* 17 (2004): 111–129.

4. Maria Pontes Ferreira and M. K. Suzy Weems, "Alcohol consumption by aging adults in the United States: Health benefits and detriments," *Journal of the American Dietetic Association* 108 (2008): 1668–1676.

5. Dana E. King, Arch G. Mainous, and Mark E. Geesey, "Adopting moderate alcohol consumption in middle age: Subsequent cardiovascular events," *American Journal of Medicine* 121 (2008): 201–206.

6. Ira J. Goldberg et al., "Wine and your heart," *Circulation* 103 (2001): 472–475.

7. Samarjit Das, Dev D. Santani, and Naranjan S. Dhalla, "Experimental evidence for the cardioprotective effects of red wine," *Experimental Clinical Cardiology* 12, no. 1 (2007): 5–10.

8. Lindsay Brown et al., "The biological responses to resveratrol and other polyphenols from alcoholic beverages," *Alcoholism: Clinical and Experimental Research* 33, no. 9 (2009): 1513–1523.

9. Cooper et al., "Wine polyphenols and promotion of cardiac health."

10. Andrew L. Waterhouse, "Wine phenolics," *Annals of the New York Academy of Science* 957 (2002): 21–36.

11. Antonia Trichopoulou, Christina Bamai, and Dimitrios Trichopoulos, "Anatomy of health effects of Mediterranean diet: Greek EPIC prospective cohort study," *British Medical Journal* 338 (2009): doi:10.1136/bmj.b2337.

12. Augusto Di Castelnuovo et al., "Alcohol dosing and total mortality in men and women, an updated meta-analysis of 34 prospective studies," *Archives of Internal Medicine* 166 (2006): 2437–2445.

13. R. Corder et al., "Red wine procyanidins and vascular health," *Nature* 444 (2006): 566.

14. Hiroki Teragawa et al., "Effect of alcohol consumption on endothelial function in men with coronary artery disease," *Atherosclerosis* 165 (2002): 145–152.

15. Romania Femia et al., "Coronary atherosclerosis and alcohol consumption: Angiographic and mortality data," *Arteriosclerosis, Thrombosis, and Vascular Biology* 26 (2006): 1607–1612.

16. Kenneth J. Mukamal et al., "Prior alcohol consumption and mortality following acute myocardial infarction," *Journal of the American Medical Association* 285 (2001): 1965–1970.

17. Michel de Lorgeril et al., "Wine drinking and risks of cardiovascular complications after recent acute myocardial infarction," *Circulation* 106 (2002): 1465–1469.

18. Augustin Scalbert and Gary Williamson, "Dietary intake and bio-availability of polyphenols," *Journal of Nutrition* 130 (2000): 2073S–2085S.

19. Guohua Cao et al., "Serum antioxidant capacity is increased by consumption of strawberries, spinach, red wine or vitamin C in elderly women," *Journal of Nutrition* 128 (1998): 2380–2390.

20. Marta Vivancos and Juan J. Moreno, "Effect of resveratrol, tyrosol and ß-sitosterol on oxidised low-density lipoprotein-simulated oxidative stress, arachidonic acid release and prostaglandin E$_2$ synthesis by RAW 264.7 macrophages," *British Journal of Nutrition* 99 (2008): 1199–1207.

21. Bianca Fuhrman, Alexandra Lavy, and Michael Aviram, "Consumption of red wine with meals reduces the susceptibility of human plasma and low-density lipoprotein to lipid peroxidation," *American Journal of Clinical Nutrition* 61 (1995): 549–554.

22. Eric B. Rimm and R. C. Ellison, "Alcohol in the Mediterranean diet," *American Journal of Clinical Nutrition* 61 (1995) (suppl.): 1378S–1382S.

23. Inder M. Singh, Medhi H. Shishehbor, and Benjamin J. Ansell, "High-density lipoprotein as a therapeutic target," *Journal of the American Medical Association* 298, no. 7 (2007) 786–798.

24. Alexandra Lavy et al., "Effect of dietary supplementation of red or white wine on human blood chemistry, hematology and coagulation: Favorable effect of red wine on plasma high-density lipoprotein," *Annals of Nutrition & Metabolism* 38 (1994): 287–294.

25. O'Keefe et al., "Alcohol and cardiovascular health."

26. Bertrand Perret et al., "Alcohol consumption is associated with enrichment of high-density lipoprotein particles in polyunsaturated lipids and increased cholesterol esterification rate," *Alcoholism: Clinical and Experimental Research* 26, no. 8 (2002): 1134–1140.

27. Pasquale Pignatelli et al., "Red and white wine differently affect collagen-induced platelet aggregation," *Pathophysiology of Haemostasis and Thrombosis* 32 (2002): 356–358.

28. Priya D. A. Issuree et al., "Resveratrol attenuates C5a-induced inflammatory responses in vitro and in vivo by inhibiting phospholipase D

and sphingosine kinase activities," *Journal of the Federation of American Societies for Experimental Biology* 23 (2009): 2412–2424.

29. Das et al., "Experimental evidence for the cardioprotective effects of red wine."

30. Tosca L. Zern and Maria Luz Fernandez, "Cardioprotective effects of dietary polyphenols," *Journal of Nutrition* 135 (2005): 2291–2294.

31. Ramon Estruch et al., "Different effects of red wine and gin consumption on inflammatory biomarkers of atherosclerosis: A prospective randomized crossover trial," *Atherosclerosis* 175 (2004): 117–123.

32. Lando L. J. Koppes et al., "Moderate alcohol consumption lowers risk of type 2 diabetes," *Diabetes Care* 28 (2005): 719–725.

33. O'Keefe et al., "Alcohol and cardiovascular health."

34. Maciej K. Malinski et al., "Alcohol consumption and cardiovascular disease mortality in hypertensive men," *Archives of Internal Medicine* 164 (2004): 623–628.

35. Goldberg et al., "Wine and your heart."

36. Paolo Gresele et al., "Resveratrol, at concentrations attainable with moderate wine consumption, stimulates human platelet nitric oxide production," *Journal of Nutrition* 138 (2008): 1602–1608.

Chapter 13

1. Norman K. Hollenberg and Naomi D. L. Fisher, "Is it the dark in dark chocolate?" *Circulation* 116 (2007): 2360–2362.

2. Roberta Lee and Michael J. Balick, "Chocolate: Healing food of the gods," *Alternative Therapies* 7, no. 5 (2001): 120–122; and Roberto Corti et al., "Cocoa and cardiovascular health," *Circulation* 119 (2009): 1433–1441.

3. Francene M. Steinberg, Monica M. Bearden, and Carl L. Keen, "Cocoa and chocolate flavonoids: Implications for cardiovascular health," *Journal of the American Dietetic Association* 103 (2003): 215–223.

4. Hollenberg and Fisher, "Is it the dark in dark chocolate?"

5. Roberto Corti, Andreas J. Flammer, Norman K. Hollenberg, and

Thomas F. Lüscher, "Cocoa and cardiovascular health," *Circulation* 119 (2009): 1433–1441.

6. Kenneth B. Miller et al., "Antioxidant activity and polyphenol and procyanidin contents of selected commercially available cocoa-containing and chocolate products in the United States," *Journal of Agricultural and Food Chemistry* 54 (2006): 4062–4068.

7. Rachel K. Johnson et al., "Dietary sugars intake and cardiovascular health: A scientific statement from the American Heart Association," *Circulation* 120 (2009): 1011–1020.

8. Mary B. Engler et al., "Flavonoid-rich dark chocolate improves endothelial function and increases plasma epicatechin concentrations in healthy adults," *Journal of the American College of Nutrition* 23, no. 3 (2004): 197–204.

9. Andreas J. Flammer et al., "Dark chocolate improves coronary vasomotion and reduces platelet reactivity," *Circulation* 116 (2007): 2376–2382.

10. Dirk Taubert, Renate Roesen, and Edgar Schömig, "Effect of cocoa and tea intake on blood pressure," *Archives of Internal Medicine* 167 (2007): 626–634.

11. Dirk Taubert et al., "Effects of low habitual cocoa intake on blood pressure and bioactive nitric oxide—a randomized controlled trial," *Journal of the American Medical Association* 298, no. 1 (2007): 49–60.

12. Taubert et al., "Effect of cocoa and tea intake on blood pressure."

13. Jan Balzer et al., "Sustained benefits in vascular function through flavonol-containing cocoa in medicated diabetic patients: A double-masked, randomized, controlled trial," *Journal of the American College of Cardiology* 51, no. 22 (2008): 2141–2149.

14. Romina di Giuseppe et al., "Regular consumption of dark chocolate is associated with low serum concentrations of C-reactive protein in a healthy Italian population," *Journal of Nutrition* 138 (2008): 1939–1945.

15. Miller et al., "Antioxidant activity and polyphenol and procyanidin contents."

16. Ibid.

Chapter 14

1. Domenico Scrutinio et al., "Physical activity for coronary heart disease; cardioprotective mechanisms and effects on prognosis," *Monaldi Archives for Chest Disease* 64 (2005): 77–87.

2. Rainer Hambrecht et al., "Effect of exercise on coronary endothelial function in patients with coronary artery disease," *New England Journal of Medicine* 342 (2000): 454–460.

3. Lyn Steffen-Batey et al., "Change in level of physical activity and risk of all-cause mortality or reinfarction: The Corpus Christi Heart Project," *Circulation* 102 (2000): 2204–2209.

4. Barry A. Franklin et al., "Safety of medically supervised cardiac rehabilitation exercise therapy: A 16-year follow-up," *Chest* 114 (1998): 902–906.

5. Paul D. Thompson, "Exercise prescription and proscription for patients with coronary artery disease," *Circulation* 112 (2005): 2354–2363.

6. Barry A. Franklin, David P. Swain, and Roy J. Shephard, "New insights in the prescription of exercise for coronary patients," *Journal of Cardiovascular Nursing* 18, no. 3 (2003): 116–123.

7. Philip A. Ades et al., "High-calorie-expenditure exercise: A new approach to cardiac rehabilitation for overweight coronary patients," *Circulation* 119 (2009): 2671–2678.

8. Thompson, "Exercise prescription and proscription for patients with coronary artery disease"; and Franklin et al., "New insights in the prescription of exercise for coronary patients."

9. M. Vona et al., "Effects of different types of exercise training followed by detraining on endothelium-dependent dilation in patients with recent myocardial infarction," *Circulation* 119 (2009): 1601–1608.

10. Peter P. Toth, "When high is low: Raising low levels of high-density lipoprotein cholesterol," *Current Cardiology Reports* 10 (2008): 488–496.

11. Juan F. Viles-Gonzalez et al., "Emerging importance of HDL cholesterol in developing high-risk coronary plaques in acute coronary syndromes," *Current Opinion in Cardiology* 18 (2003): 286–294.

12. Scrutinio et al., "Physical activity for coronary heart disease."

13. Domenico Lapenna et al., "Glutathione-related antioxidant defenses in human atherosclerotic plaques," *Circulation* 97 (1998): 1930–1934.

14. Christian K. Roberts and R. James Barnard, "Effects of exercise and diet on chronic disease," *Journal of Applied Physiology* 98 (2005): 3–30.

15. Ulrich Förstermann and Thomas Münzel, "Endothelial nitric oxide synthase in vascular disease: From marvel to menace," *Circulation* 113 (2006): 1708–1714.

16. Jean Davignon and Peter Ganz, "Role of endothelial dysfunction in atherosclerosis," *Circulation* 109 (2004): III-27–III-32.

17. Arthur S. Leon et al., "Cardiac rehabilitation and secondary prevention of coronary heart disease: An American Heart Association scientific statement from the Council on Clinical Cardiology (Subcommittee on Exercise, Cardiac Rehabilitation, and Prevention) and the Council on Nutrition, Physical Activity, and Metabolism (Subcommittee on Physical Activity), in collaboration with the American Association of Cardiovascular and Pulmonary Rehabilitation," *Circulation* 111 (2005): 369–376.

18. Pedro Zaros et al., "Effect of 6 months of physical exercise on the nitrate/nitrite levels in hypertensive postmenopausal women," *BMC Women's Health* 9 (2009): doi:10.1186/1472-6874-9-17.

19. Department of Health and Human Services, National Institutes of Health, National Heart, Lung and Blood Institute, "Calculate your body mass index," http://www.nhlbisupport.com/bmi/.

20. Roberts and Barnard, "Effects of exercise and diet on chronic disease."

Index

About the Author

JANET BOND BRILL grew up in New York City, the daughter of a prominent actor and a psychoanalyst. She graduated from the Walden School in Manhattan and earned a B.S. in biology, as well as both a master's degree and a doctoral degree in exercise physiology, at the University of Miami. She also holds a second master's degree in nutrition science from Florida International University. She is a registered dietitian, certified personal trainer, and certified wellness coach.

The author of *Cholesterol Down: 10 Simple Steps to Lower Your Cholesterol in 4 Weeks Without Prescription Drugs,* Dr. Brill has also been published in noted scientific journals including the *International Journal of Sport Nutrition,* the *International Journal of Obesity,* and the *American Journal of Lifestyle Medicine,* and published and quoted in leading consumer publications including *Shape, Prevention,* and *Men's Health.* She is a frequent professional speaker, a nutrition expert on national television, and maintains a private nutrition consulting practice. Dr. Brill also serves as director of nutrition for Fitness Together, the world's largest franchise of personal trainers.

Dr. Brill practices what she preaches, having completed four marathons and countless road races, many for charitable causes. Dr. Brill enjoys spending her free time with her husband, Sam; her three children; and her golden retriever, Simba.

Also by Dr. Janet Brill

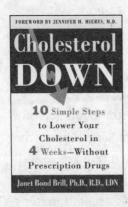

IF YOU ARE ONE of the nearly 100 million Americans struggling with high cholesterol, then Dr. Janet Brill offers you a revolutionary new plan for taking control of your health—without the risks of statin drugs. With Dr. Brill's breakthrough Cholesterol Down Plan, you simply add nine "miracle foods" to your regular diet and thirty minutes of walking to your daily routine. This straightforward and easy-to-follow program can lower your LDL ("bad") cholesterol by as much as 47 percent in just four weeks. Live your healthiest life with Dr. Brill's plan, a safe and effective alternative to statin drugs.

Cholesterol Down
*Ten Simple Steps to Lower Your Cholesterol
in Four Weeks—Without Prescription Drugs*
$14.00 (Canada:$17.99)
978-0-307-33911-9